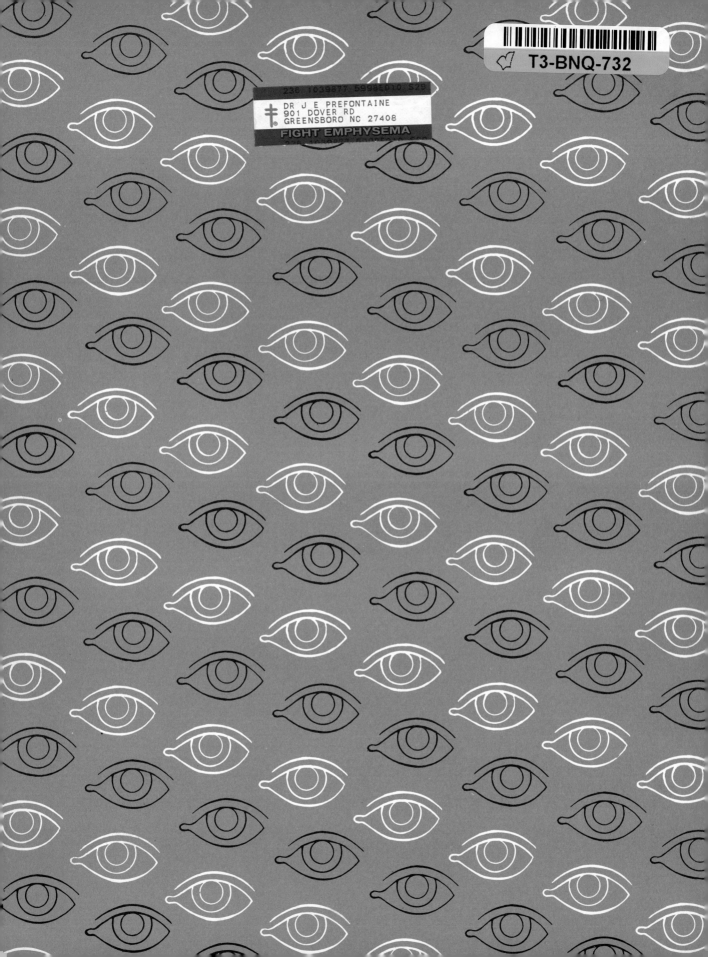

AN ATLAS OF
Diseases of the Eye

First published . . January 1957

Reprinted . . . . October 1957

AN ATLAS OF

Diseases of the Eye

Compiled by

E. S. PERKINS, M.B., F.R.C.S.

Reader in Ophthalmology, Institute of Ophthalmology
University of London

and

PETER HANSELL, M.R.C.S., F.R.P.S.

Director, Departments of Illustration and Photography
Westminster Medical School and Institute of Ophthalmology
University of London

With a foreword by

SIR STEWART DUKE-ELDER

K.C.V.O., M.A., D.Sc., Ph.D., M.D., F.R.C.S.

Little, Brown & Company
Boston
1957

This book has been printed in England by
W. S. Cowell Limited at their Press in the
Butter Market, Ipswich. The text has been set
in 10pt Plantin, with subheadings in 10pt and
page titles in 18pt Condensed Sans Serif No.
14. The introductory matter is set in Perpetua.
Reproduction is by eight-colour photolitho-
graphy on Gateway Twinprint Cartridge paper

Published simultaneously in Canada by Little, Brown
& Company (Canada) Limited. Published in Great
Britain by J. & A. Churchill Limited, London

Foreword

There is no doubt that the only satisfactory way to learn medicine is by the repeated study day after day and month after month of large numbers of patients in a hospital under the guidance of a wise teacher. Thus the student first finds his way around the medical world; but as speciality succeeds speciality in the medical curriculum and when studentship is transformed into practice, the distinctness of the memory of clinical pictures necessarily becomes blurred. Particularly is this so in a subject such as ophthalmology, for in most medical schools the study of diseases of the eye receives less attention than it deserves, crowded out as it is by the multitude of subjects which appear to have greater immediate interest. This is indeed unfortunate – to the general practitioner, because the importance of recognizing ocular conditions in general practice is often crucial, particularly the differentiation of what is trivial from what may be of serious import; and to the specialist in many fields, as well as to the general practitioner, in so far as an understanding of vascular and other changes as seen in the eye, is frequently of immense value in establishing the diagnosis and assessing the prognosis of a host of general systemic diseases.

How is the position most easily remedied? There is no doubt that a pictorial representation of pathological conditions is much more meaningful and valuable for this purpose than a host of printed words, and an Atlas supplemented by a text the best substitute for the patient himself. This volume, much of which has previously been published in the form of booklets, is an attempt to fulfil this want, to provide the student, the general practitioner and the non-ophthalmological specialist with a short guide to the more common and important ocular disorders. For this purpose no trouble has been spared.

All the illustrations have been specially selected or prepared in order that a representative collection could be made widely available. In the case of fundus appearances use has been made of both colour photography and drawing; the selective hand of the artist serves to underline the important features of any given condition, whereas photography more nearly reproduces a single ophthalmoscopic view with its profusion of distracting detail: some care in interpretation is therefore necessary.

The external appearances have mainly been recorded in colour by the camera, supplemented where necessary by the artist whose particular contribution is in the synthesis of microscopic views seen by slit-lamp illumination. Particular attention has also been paid to the photo-mechanical method of reproducing the originals, and by means of offset lithography the ideal has largely been attained.

There is no doubt that the excellence of modern techniques of reproduction makes many of these conditions live. But these techniques are expensive; and the cost of an Atlas of this type, if it were to be published at its economic price would be prohibitive. Its publication, however, at a relatively low cost, has been made possible by the generosity and public spirit of the firm of Roche Products Limited. One of the features of modern medicine is the partnership that is nowadays frequently formed between it and the large pharmaceutical firms, many of which have done much to further the therapeutic aspects of medicine by the immense effort they expend in research and the happy collaboration they offer to academic laboratories; the subsidy of an Atlas of this type by Roche Products Limited so that it may become available to the profession at about one-tenth of its cost price is a novel contribution to the dissemination of knowledge. For this, and in so far as the Atlas may aid in the treatment of our patients, we are grateful to them.

INSTITUTE OF OPHTHALMOLOGY,   STEWART DUKE-ELDER
UNIVERSITY OF LONDON.

Acknowledgements

It is clear that a compilation of this character can never be complete and must always depend to some extent upon the willing co-operation of many people.

In particular, members of the medical staff of Moorfields Eye Hospital (incorporating the Royal London Eye Hospital, the Royal Westminster Ophthalmic Hospital and the Central London Ophthalmic Hospital) have made the greatest contribution by making their records so freely available. Dr Norman Ashton of the Institute of Ophthalmology has been kind enough to provide pathological material to supplement purely clinical appearances and Mr E. F. Fincham was responsible for producing the special cataract photograph. Certain gaps have been nobly filled by other hospitals including Guy's Hospital, St Bartholomew's Hospital, Westminster Hospital and the Hospital for Sick Children, London. Mr D. P. Greaves of University College Hospital has also been most helpful in providing specific examples required for this atlas.

Most of the pictures themselves have been prepared by the staff of the Medical Illustration Department of the Institute of Ophthalmology amongst whom we are pleased to name Mr N. Jeffreys, F.I.B.P., and Mr T. R. Tarrant, M.M.A.A. The work of other illustrators is also represented and we are glad to acknowledge the following: Miss J. Trotman, Mr E. R. Alexander, Mr A. W. Head, Mrs L. Geddes and Theodore Hamblin, Ltd.

The task of preparing the manuscript for publication has fallen to Miss J. Richards and Miss B. Bate. This work has involved many revisions and their help in this respect has been invaluable. Miss M. H. T. Yuille has also kindly assisted in checking proofs.

We should like to thank Sir Stewart Duke-Elder who was responsible for the original plan; both he and Mr R. C. Davenport have made many helpful suggestions at various stages of production. Mr Frank Law and Mr E. F. King have both carefully appraised the pictures and text; as a result of their helpful criticisms several changes have been made.

Special equipment has been used in production of many of the illustrations and reference should be made to Messrs Clement Clarke Ltd, for making certain technical facilities available to us.

More than a word of recognition is due to the printers – Messrs W. S. Cowell Ltd of Ipswich. They have lavished unusual care and attention on the reproduction of originals which, in many instances, contained very fine detail. So much has depended on their efforts and the consistent results which they have obtained from different types of material are a singular achievement.

Lastly, we should like to thank Roche Products Limited for their generous support and co-operation throughout the preparation of the volume.

E.S.P.
P.H.

CONTENTS

PART IV *The Fundus in Systemic Disease*

PART V *The Fundus in Local Disease*

The Normal Eye

ALTHOUGH A DETAILED KNOWLEDGE of the normal anatomy of the eye and orbit is not necessary for an understanding of most of the conditions illustrated in this Atlas, some reminder of the gross anatomy and its terminology may be helpful as an introduction.

The Eyelids   The eyelids consist essentially of a plate of condensed fibrous tissue (the tarsal plate) lined internally by conjunctiva and covered externally by the orbicularis muscle and skin. The Meibomian glands are embedded in the tarsal plate and open on the free margin of the lid very close to its posterior border.

The palpebral fissure is the almond-shaped space formed when the lids are open. It will be seen from Fig. 1 that normally the upper lid cuts across the upper part of the cornea, while the lower lid margin is related to the junction between cornea and sclera – the limbus.

The inner and outer angles of the palpebral fissure are known as the inner and outer canthi and at the inner canthus can be seen the caruncle and plica semilunaris. On the lid margin by the plica semilunaris is a small elevation known as the papilla lacrimalis in the centre of which is a hole, the punctum lacrimalis through which the tears flow. The punctum lies in close apposition to the globe and cannot normally be seen unless the lid is everted.

The Globe   The eyeball is so positioned in the orbit that the anterior surface of the cornea is just in line with the superior and inferior orbital margins – a useful relation in the assessment of proptosis.

The cornea joins the sclera at the limbus, the corneal epithelium becoming continuous with the epithelium of the conjunctiva which is adherent here to the underlying episcleral tissue. Elsewhere the conjunctiva forms a loose covering for the globe and extends peripherally to form two pockets – the upper and lower fornices, before continuing on to the posterior surface of the lids (Fig. 3).

The anterior chamber is the space enclosed by the cornea anteriorly and the lens and iris posteriorly. The pupillary margin of the iris is in constant contact with the anterior surface of the lens, although aqueous humour is able to flow from the posterior chamber (the small space between the periphery of the iris and the lens) through the pupil into the anterior chamber, from which it drains through the trabeculae into Schlemm's canal.

The iris, ciliary body and choroid form a continuous structure called the uveal tract which is derived embryologically in part from the anterior portion of the optic cup and in part from the surrounding mesoderm.

The choroid is a purely vascular structure which supplies the outer one-third of the retina with blood. Fig. 3 is a diagrammatic sagittal section through the eye and orbit, showing the gross relations of the bony orbit, lids, globe and intra-ocular structures.

The Slit-Lamp Microscope   Several conditions in this Atlas are illustrated by drawings of slit-lamp appearances and for those unfamiliar with the apparatus a brief description is included here.

The instrument consists of two parts; a low-power binocular microscope mounted horizontally and an illumination system which provides a bright slit of variable width focusing sharply at the point of focus of the microscope. It is designed primarily to examine the transparent media of the eye; i.e. the cornea, aqueous humour, lens and vitreous. The narrow slit beam gives the effect of an optical section in transparent or semi-transparent structures and clearly demonstrates differences in optical density due to anatomical structure or pathological change.

As can be seen in the drawing of a normal eye (Fig. 4) the anterior and posterior surfaces of the cornea show clearly, the corneal stroma reflects some light but the normal aqueous humour is optically empty. The anterior surface of the lens shows well and the discontinuity of the layers of the lens substance can be seen.

I

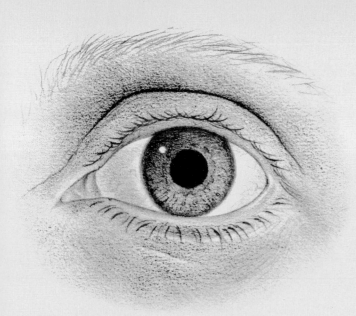

1

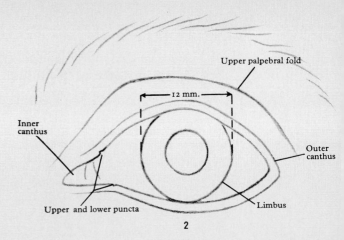

Inner canthus

Upper palpebral fold

12 mm.

Outer canthus

Upper and lower puncta

Limbus

2

FIG. 1. ⎫
FIG. 2. ⎬ EXTERNAL APPEARANCE OF NORMAL EYE

FIG. 3. SAGITTAL SECTION THROUGH ORBIT

FIG. 4. THE EYE AS SEEN BY SLIT-LAMP ILLUMINATION

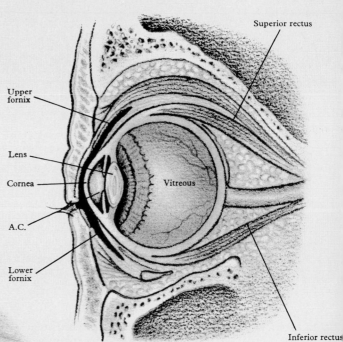

Superior rectus

Upper fornix

Lens

Cornea

Vitreous

A.C.

Lower fornix

Inferior rectus

3

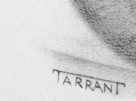

TARRANT

4

Congenital Defects of Lids and Orbit

Coloboma of the Lids A notch in the lid margin is not uncommonly found as a congenital defect. Although the term coloboma is used to describe this condition, it is in no way analogous to the coloboma found in the iris or choroid and described later in this series. The defect may appear as a small notch in the upper lid margin or may extend to involve the whole thickness of the lid, as can be seen in Fig. 1. This photograph also shows the corneal scarring which may occur due to the exposure of the cornea by the lid defect. The pathogenesis of the condition is not entirely clear, as in no stage of development does the lid normally have a cleft. It seems probable that the defect is due to pressure of amniotic bands during development of the embryo.

Epicanthus The term epicanthus is used to describe the vertical skin folds at the inner canthi, seen in the photograph, Fig. 2. Such folds are normal during foetal development from the third to the sixth month but, in the Caucasian races, they have normally disappeared by birth. In the Mongolian races, on the other hand, the condition persists into adult life, giving rise to the typical Mongolian eye. When it persists in the Caucasian races the child is seen to have a broad flat nose with widely separated eyes and often an apparent convergent squint. Careful examination, however, will show that the eyes are actually straight and the epicanthal folds and the apparent squint can frequently be made to disappear by pinching up the loose skin over the bridge of the nose. Many mild cases cure themselves when the nose develops normally at puberty or before. In more severe cases operative procedures are necessary to remove the skin folds.

Ptosis A drooping lid on one or both sides is a common congenital defect. The degree of ptosis varies from a hardly perceptible narrowing of the palpebral fissure to a complete paralysis of elevation of the upper lid, which hangs down obscuring the pupil, Fig. 3. The patient attempts to remedy the condition by raising the eyebrow, by contracting the frontalis muscle and tilting the head back, producing a very typical appearance. The absence or weakness of the levator palpebrae superioris muscle, which is the cause of the ptosis, may be associated with weakness or absence of the superior rectus muscle as evidenced by poor elevation of the globe on the affected side.

Dysostosis of the Skull There are several conditions in which too early fusion of the cranial sutures results in deformities of the skull. Oxycephaly, Crouzon's disease and hypertelorism are clearly recognizable clinical types and a photograph (Fig. 4) of a child with oxycephaly has been chosen to represent the group. The abnormal development of the orbits causes proptosis, and stretching of the optic nerve may result in papilloedema and optic atrophy, causing defective vision.

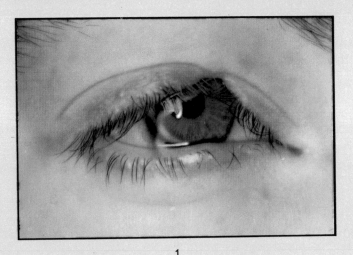

1

FIG. I.   COLOBOMA OF THE LID WITH CORNEAL SCARRING

FIG. 2.   EPICANTHUS

FIG. 3.   CONGENITAL PTOSIS

FIG. 4.   OXYCEPHALY

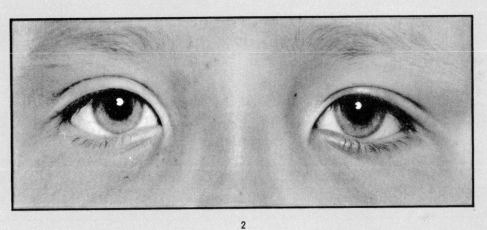

2

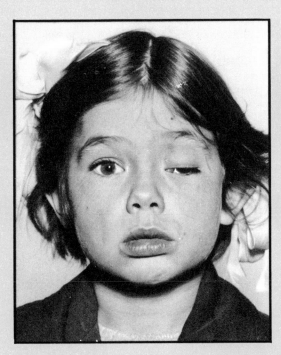

3

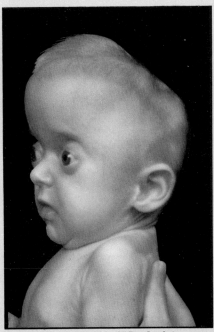

(Hospital for Sick Children, London)

4

Inflammatory Lesions of the Lids

Hordeolum or Stye This well known and common condition is essentially a staphylococcal infection of a lash follicle and corresponds to a boil of the skin elsewhere. It starts as a painful swelling of the whole lid so that at first it may be difficult to find a localized lesion, but soon one area becomes more swollen and, as pus forms, a yellow point associated with an eyelash can be seen near the lid margin, Fig. 1.

The differential diagnosis is from an acute inflammation of the Meibomian glands – the so-called hordeolum internum. A stye is in the skin and always associated with the lashes, while a Meibomian infection is in the tarsal plate and the skin is not primarily involved. Examination of the conjunctival surface of the lid in hordeolum internum will show a red velvety area with a central yellow spot, through which pus will later discharge. As the Meibomian glands are embedded in tough fibrous tissue, pain and reaction may be more severe than in an ordinary stye. These acute infections of the lid may be associated with acne, general debility or such conditions as diabetes.

Local treatment is by heat until the abscess points, when it may be opened to allow drainage of the pus. Removal of the affected lash is frequently sufficient in a hordeolum externum. If the infection is severe, systemic treatment with antibiotics should be considered.

Chalazion This is a chronic affection of the Meibomian glands. A painless firm lump appears in the lid and slowly increases in size, Fig. 2. Symptoms are few, although occasionally pressure on the cornea may produce some astigmatism.

Frequently called a Meibomian cyst it is, however, not truly cystic but a chronic granuloma caused primarily by the retention of the secretion of the gland. The skin moves freely over the swelling and if the lid is everted a grey spot surrounded by inflamed conjunctiva will be seen at the site of the lesion. Treatment is incision and curettage through the conjunctival surface of the lid.

Blepharitis Chronic inflammation of the lid margins is a very common and distressing condition. The inflammation may be mild and consist simply in a hyperaemia of the lid margin with scaling of the skin (squamous blepharitis) or more severe and affect the lash follicles, leading to destruction or distortion of the lashes and deformity of the lid margin (ulcerative blepharitis).

Both types are commonly associated with seborrhoea of the skin. Attention to the general health is of great importance in the treatment and local applications to the lids will not prevent recurrence unless the underlying cause is removed. Fig. 3 shows a long-standing case of ulcerative blepharitis in which the lid margins are deformed, many lashes are missing and others are distorted and turn in to rub on the cornea.

Acute Dacryocystitis Although acute inflammation of the lacrimal sac is not a lid condition it has been included here because it may have to be considered in the differential diagnosis of inflammatory swellings at the inner canthus.

Acute dacryocystitis may be an incident in chronic infection of the lacrimal sac or may be an initial infection. Fig. 4 shows the typical appearance of the swelling below the medial canthal ligament. Lacrimal drainage is blocked, thus causing epiphora. Pressure over the sac (if this is not too painful) may cause regurgitation of pus through the puncta.

Treatment consists of local heat and systemic antibiotics but incision may be required.

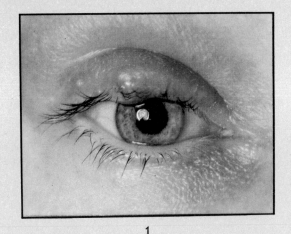

1

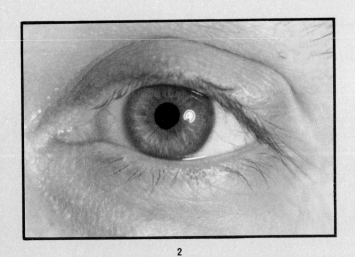

2

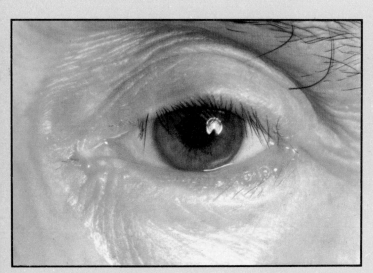

3

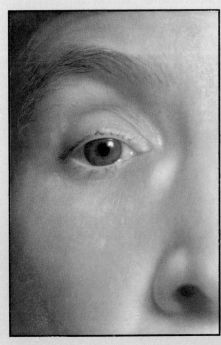

4

FIG. 1.   STYE (HORDEOLUM EXTERNUM)

FIG. 2.   CHALAZION

FIG. 3.   ULCERATIVE BLEPHARITIS

FIG. 4.   ACUTE DACRYOCYSTITIS

Neoplasms of the Lids

Benign Simple papillomata, particularly along the lid margin as shown in Fig. 1, are common on the lids but require no special treatment except excision for cosmetic reasons. Haemangiomata are less common but of more interest; they are sometimes accompanied by meningeal lesions while a choroidal angioma may occur with other congenital abnormalities of the eyes, causing buphthalmos or infantile glaucoma. Fig. 2 illustrates the typical 'port wine stain' due to a capillary angioma.

Cavernous haemangiomata may occur in the lids and give rise to bluish soft swellings which can be reduced by pressure over them. They are congenital but tend to grow rapidly in the first four years of life and may cause ptosis or exophthalmos. Treatment is by surgical excision, the insertion of radon seeds or the injection of sclerosing fluids into the vessels.

Malignant The lids and skin of the nose near the inner canthus are very common sites for the development of carcinoma in older people. Basal-celled carcinomata or rodent ulcers are more common than the squamous epitheliomata and are characterized histologically by downgrowths of solid darkly staining cells into the dermis. Clinically a rodent ulcer starts as a small nodule in the skin which gradually enlarges and breaks down to form an ulcer with an indurated base and rolled edges. Bleeding from the ulcer is common but any skin nodule which has been present for several months in a patient over the age of forty should be viewed with suspicion. Early removal may save the otherwise inevitable growth of the tumour with much destruction of the lid tissues. However, in the case of large tumours, irradiation may be preferable as excision would leave too big a defect in the lid.

Fig. 3 is a photograph of a typical basal-celled carcinoma of the lower lid. The rolled edges and breaking down base of the ulcer can be clearly seen.

The treatment of choice is excision of the tumour, for although rodent ulcers are very sensitive to irradiation there is some danger to the eye or lacrimal passages in irradiating the lids.

Squamous-celled carcinoma is less common than rodent ulcer but tends to be more malignant and may metastasize to the lymph nodes in the pre-auricular or the submaxillary region. Histologically the tumour shows more resemblance to the general structure of the epidermis. Well-developed prickle cells surround areas of squamous cells which undergo their normal degeneration to form cell nests of acid-staining cornified epithelial cells.

Clinically it appears either as an ulcerated area less symmetrical than a rodent ulcer or as a papillomatous growth. Local extension occurs slowly but relentlessly, eating away the lids, the soft structures of the orbit and even the bone itself if the tumour is left untreated.

Fig. 4 shows a squamous-celled carcinoma which has destroyed a considerable amount of the tissue of the lower lid; in such cases plastic surgery is required to fill in the defect after excision of the growth. Such cases illustrate the importance of early diagnosis and treatment of malignant neoplasms of the lid.

Treatment is the same as that for rodent ulcer, particular care being taken to remove the whole tumour, as the mortality rate is appreciable. Careful follow-up examination is necessary for many years.

7

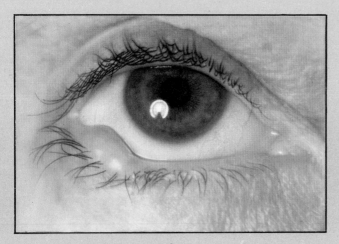

1

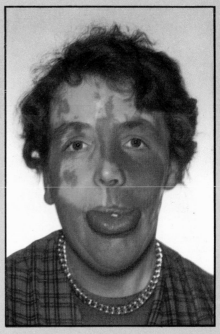

2

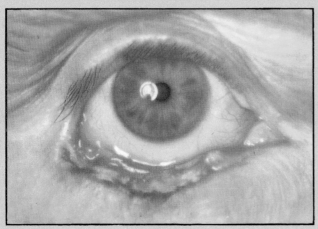

3

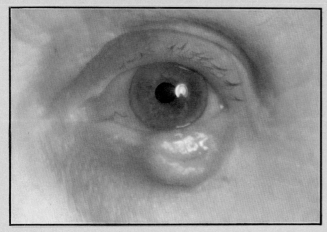

4

FIG. 1. SIMPLE PAPILLOMA OF THE LID

FIG. 2. NAEVUS FLAMMEUS

FIG. 3. RODENT ULCER

FIG. 4. EPITHELIOMA

Skin Conditions

ALMOST ANY SKIN CONDITION may affect the lids but only those in which the region of the eyelids is primarily involved or which have particular ocular significance will be discussed and illustrated here.

Contact Dermatitis This very common condition may follow the topical application of drugs, cosmetics or any foreign material. It is of particular importance in ophthalmology in which the continued use of drops and ointments frequently causes an allergic reaction in a sensitive patient. Penicillin ointment applied to the lids and atropine drops very commonly cause such irritation.

The changes in the skin are essentially eczematous in nature and usually arise after repeated use of the agent. Itching is a prominent symptom and the skin of the lids, particularly the lower lid, becomes red and scaly, and in severe cases the inflammation may spread over the whole face.

Fig. 1 illustrates a case of contact dermatitis following the use of eye-drops. The lids are swollen and the skin shows vesiculation extending well beyond the lids, an appearance which always suggests a drug reaction.

Herpes Ophthalmicus Herpes zoster involving the ophthalmic division of the trigeminal nerve is of particular importance in ophthalmology. The history of onset with pain and constitutional disturbance followed by erythema and vesicle formation is characteristic. The lesions may occur in the area of distribution of the whole of the ophthalmic division of the trigeminal nerve or a part only. The frontal branch is always involved but it is when the lacrimal and nasociliary branches are also affected that corneal involvement and iritis are likely to occur. It is a good working rule that if the side of the tip of the nose is involved, eye complications are likely. The corneal and uveal complications will be discussed in later sections. Fig. 2 shows the typical distribution and appearance of the vesicles. The frontal branch of the trigeminal nerve is mainly affected in this case.

Xanthelasma The skin of the lids, particularly towards the inner canthus, is a common site for the deposition of lipoid material. Fig. 3 shows the typical yellowish, soft plaques. Xanthelasma affects women more frequently than men and it may be associated with a hyperlipaemia. It causes no symptoms but may require excision for cosmetic reasons.

Acne Rosacea This common skin disease is frequently associated with a blepharo-conjunctivitis and sometimes a keratitis. The typical flushing of the skin of the cheeks (Fig. 4) often extends to the lids, causing a scaly desquamation and diffuse hyperaemia. The conjunctiva shows engorgement of the vessels with some hypersecretion. The condition is not serious unless or until the cornea is affected.

9

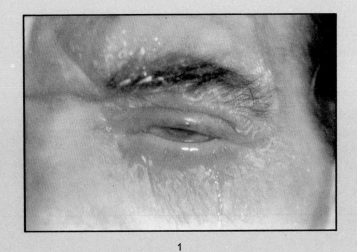

1

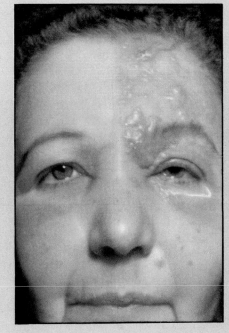

2

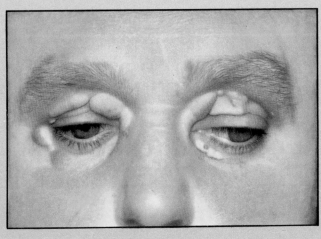

3

FIG. 1.   CONTACT DERMATITIS

FIG. 2.   HERPES OPHTHALMICUS

FIG. 3.   XANTHELASMA

FIG. 4.   ROSACEA

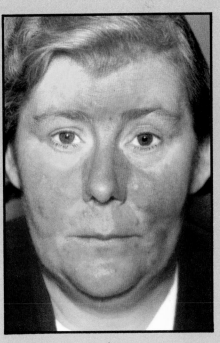

4

Ectropion and Entropion

MALPOSITIONS OF THE LID are common in elderly people and although not serious in themselves, give rise to considerable discomfort and irritation.

Ectropion This is a condition in which the lower lid falls away from the globe and becomes everted. The drainage of tears takes place mainly through the lower punctum and unless this is in close apposition to the globe it is unable to function and epiphora results. The constant flow of tears over the lid, combined with wiping the eye with a handkerchief, causes excoriation and subsequent retraction of the skin, tending to aggravate the eversion.

Ectropion may be caused by scarring of the skin, as for example following irradiation of a rodent ulcer, or more commonly through a lessening of muscle tone combined with a decrease in orbital fat in old people which allows the lower lid to fall away from the globe. There may be some spastic element present also – the lower fibres of the orbicularis muscle contracting more than the fibres near the lid margin, thus tending to cause eversion of the lid.

Figs 1 and 2 are photographs of typical senile ectropion. The conjunctival surface of the lid is exposed and the punctum is well away from the globe. The skin at the inner canthus is excoriated and taut, pulling the lid downwards. The exposed conjunctiva becomes chronically inflamed and unsightly. In the earliest stages massage of the lid and the use of a bland ointment on the skin may alleviate the condition but usually some plastic procedure is necessary to bring the lid back into its normal position. Fig. 3 shows an ectropion caused by scarring and contracture of the skin.

Entropion In entropion the lid turns inwards and the lashes cause much irritation by rubbing on the cornea. Unlike ectropion it may affect either the upper or lower lid. Again the causes are scarring, this time of the tarsal plate, and senile changes of muscle-tone in which the marginal fibres of the orbicularis contract more strongly than the peripheral fibres, thus turning the lid inwards. The latter condition of senile spastic entropion is much more common in this country than the cicatricial entropion of the upper lid following such diseases as trachoma, in which the tarsal plate is severely scarred and buckled.

Spastic entropion is only present intermittently at first but can be elicited by asking the patient to squeeze the eyes tightly shut, when, on subsequent opening, the lower lid will be seen to be turned inwards. This is well shown in Fig. 4. A slight pull on the skin of the lid will replace it to its normal position. After a while the lid becomes inverted more frequently and corneal ulceration from the abrasions caused by the lashes may result.

As a temporary expedient, strips of sticking plaster can be used to draw down the skin of the lid but operative procedures designed to strengthen the lower fibres of the orbicularis or weaken the marginal fibres are normally necessary.

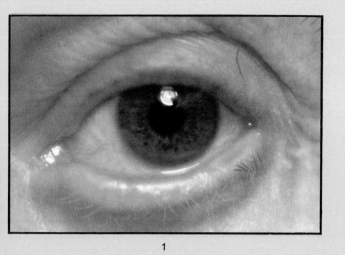

1

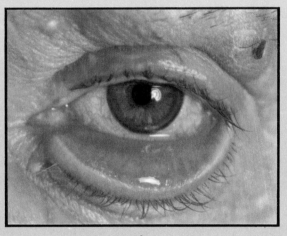

2

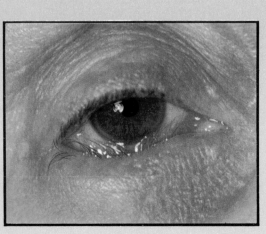

3

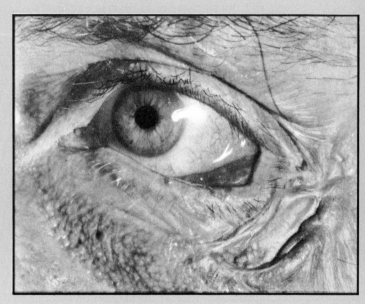

4

FIG. 1.   SENILE ECTROPION

FIG. 2.   A MORE ADVANCED STAGE

FIG. 3.   CICATRICIAL ECTROPION

FIG. 4.   SPASTIC ENTROPION

Exophthalmos

BILATERAL EXOPHTHALMOS is usually associated with endocrine disorders, while unilateral cases are most often due to local disease in the orbit.

Endocrine Exophthalmos The association between disease of the thyroid gland and exophthalmos has been recognized for over a hundred years but although the clinical picture is so characteristic, the underlying pathology is still not clear. Briefly, two syndromes can be distinguished. First, a slight exophthalmos with marked lid retraction occurring in thyrotoxicosis, and secondly, a more severe proptosis frequently associated with ophthalmoplegia, which may follow thyroidectomy or may occur *ab initio* in patients with normal or subnormal thyroid activity.

The staring appearance of patients with Graves's disease is so well known as to require little description except to emphasize that the actual protrusion of the eyes is usually small and the appearance is largely due to the lid retraction. Fig. 1 is a photograph of such a patient, showing how the upper lid is raised to expose the sclera above the cornea. In the majority of cases the ocular condition improves when the thyroid over-activity has been reduced either by medical or surgical treatment. Any remaining disfigurement can be overcome by a small lateral tarsorrhaphy.

The much more serious condition of exophthalmos with ophthalmoplegia occasionally follows thyroidectomy and is thought to be due to an excess of pituitary hormone, the excretion of which is no longer held in check when the thyroid activity is rapidly reduced. The disease may also occur spontaneously in a rather later age-group than thyrotoxicosis, and in contrast to the latter it affects men more often than women.

Oedema of the lids, diplopia and prominence of one, and later both eyes, are the initial symptoms. The protrusion is much greater than the exophthalmos of Graves's disease and in severe cases may become so extreme that the lids are unable to close over the eye and corneal ulceration, perforation and loss of the eye may result unless treatment is prompt and energetic. Lid retraction may be present but is not universal as in thyrotoxicosis. Paralysis of elevation is the most marked defect but all movements are usually restricted. Fig. 2 shows the gross proptosis with oedema of the lids and folds of protruding chemotic conjunctiva. A tarsorrhaphy has been performed on the right side to protect the cornea.

The condition may progress very rapidly, particularly in post-operative cases, but more commonly a chronic state of exophthalmos and ophthalmoplegia ensues. The cornea must be protected at all costs and if tarsorrhaphy fails, orbital decompression is necessary.

Exophthalmos due to Orbital Lesions Any space-occupying lesion in the orbit may produce proptosis of the eye. Haemorrhage, inflammation, aneurysms and new growths of the optic nerve or orbital contents are the most common causes.

Apart from the traumatic or infective group, the history of onset is of gradual prominence of one eye which may be displaced forward in the direction of the optic axis or to one side, depending on the position of the tumour. Vision is only affected early in neoplasms of the optic nerve but diplopia will arise if the movements of the eye are limited in any way. Fig. 3 shows a case of proptosis due to an orbital neoplasm.

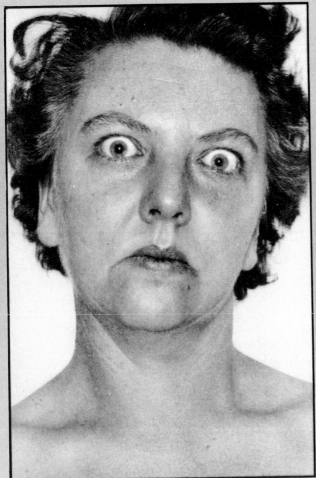

(Westminster Hospital, London)

1

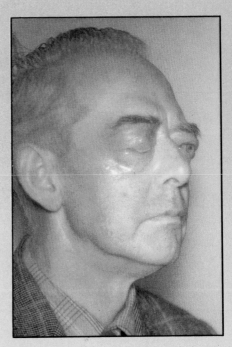

2

FIG. 1.   THYROTOXICOSIS WITH MARKED LID RETRACTION AND SLIGHT EXOPHTHALMOS

FIG. 2.   THYROTROPIC EXOPHTHALMOS

FIG. 3.   PROPTOSIS DUE TO ORBITAL NEOPLASM

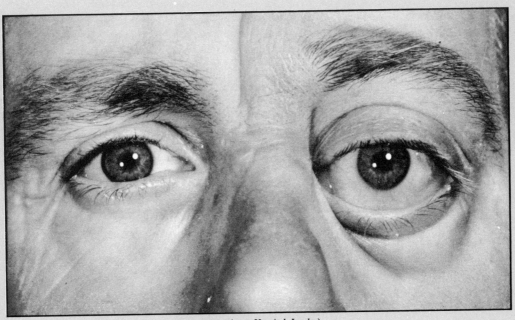

(Westminster Hospital, London)

3

Miscellaneous Conditions of the Lids

Marginal Cysts The glands of Moll are sweat glands occurring in the lid margin associated with the lashes and not uncommonly they become blocked to form cystic swellings. These have a predilection for the lower lid near the lacrimal punctum as illustrated in Fig. 1.

Sebaceous cysts occur in the lids as elsewhere in the skin. They may arise from the glands of Zeis, which are sebaceous glands associated with the lashes, producing a similar appearance to the sweat gland cyst illustrated in Fig. 1. The contents, however, are composed of epithelial cells, fatty granules and cholesterol crystals as opposed to the clear fluid in the cysts of Moll's glands. Treatment is excision of the cyst.

Oedema of the Lids The thin skin and loose subcutaneous tissue of the lids predisposes to oedema in this region. Local inflammations, angioneurotic oedema, renal disease, myxoedema and parasitic infestation with trypanosomiasis and trichiniasis (in which marked swelling of the lids is an important symptom) are some of the many causes.

In myxoedema the swelling is not a true oedema and does not pit on pressure. The puffy lids with the dry skin and sparse eyebrows help to give the characteristic facies of the disease. An advanced case is illustrated in Fig. 2. In this patient the left eye is severely affected and ptosis has resulted from the swelling and weight of the upper lid.

Dacryoadenitis Inflammations of the lacrimal gland are comparatively rare and most of the cases which do occur involve children or young adolescents. Acute dacryoadenitis may occur as a complication of mumps and, more rarely, of other acute infections. A painful swelling appears in the upper lid, causing some degree of ptosis, Fig. 3. On raising the lid the swollen palpebral portion of the gland can be seen bulging beneath the conjunctiva, Fig. 4.

Vaccinia Accidental infection of the lids with vaccinia may occur as an auto-inoculation or from contact with a vaccinated person. The pustule so formed takes the typical course but, owing to the loose tissue of the lid, local swelling is marked. The pre-auricular lymph nodes are enlarged and constitutional disturbances such as fever and malaise develop about the eighth day.

Fig. 5 shows vaccinia pustules on the left lower lid and right cheek of a young girl. The scabs eventually fall off, leaving a red pitted scar which slowly becomes white and atrophic.

More rarely vaccinial lesions on the lid margin may spread to the palpebral conjunctiva and even involve the cornea.

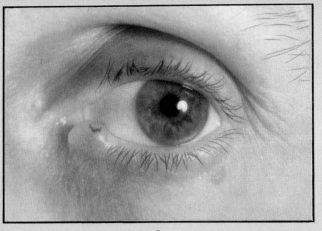

1

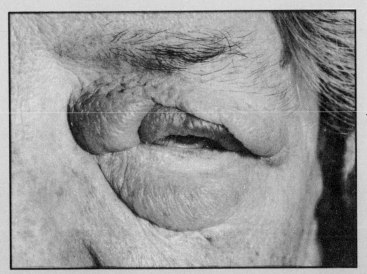

2

3

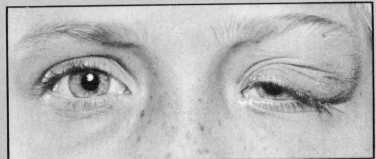

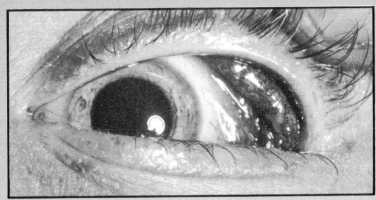

4

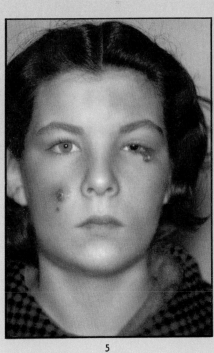

5

Inflammations of the Conjunctiva

THE DIFFERENTIAL DIAGNOSIS of a 'red eye' is a common clinical problem and it is usual to divide the type of injection into conjunctival or ciliary. By this is meant that when the vessels supplying the conjunctiva only are dilated the redness is superficial and more marked towards the fornices, but when the deeper vessels which enter the eye to supply the cornea and ciliary body are dilated the redness is less bright in colour and is situated particularly in the limbal area surrounding the cornea. There are, however, some branches from the deeper vessels which supply the conjunctiva at the limbus and these may also become dilated in an inflammation of the conjunctiva. It follows that the distinction between the two types of injection is not as clear-cut as is sometimes suggested, but as demonstrated in Fig. 1, the majority of cases of simple conjunctivitis show the typical 'conjunctival' type of injection. Not infrequently, however, a conjunctival inflammation is associated with a superficial keratitis and in these cases the injection will always extend to the limbal vessels. Fig. 2 is a photograph of a case of kerato-conjunctivitis in which the corneal lesion has been stained with fluorescein.

Acute catarrhal conjunctivitis Acute catarrhal conjunctivitis as illustrated in Fig. 1 may be caused by a variety of organisms and is characterized by conjunctival injection and a muco-purulent discharge. Provided the eye is not bandaged the condition tends to recover spontaneously, a tendency which can be hastened by an appropriate antibiotic drug applied locally.

Tuberculosis of the conjunctiva in contrast to acute catarrhal conjunctivitis, is a chronic infection which may take many different forms. Hypertrophic, nodular and ulcerative lesions are the most common manifestations but all types tend to run a long course with little evidence of spontaneous remission. The advent of streptomycin has, however, very favourably influenced the prognosis.

Fig. 3 is a photograph of a tuberculous lesion of the palpebral conjunctiva, nodular in type, which would probably have progressed to ulceration if left untreated.

Follicular conjunctivitis The two conditions described above are both examples of a bacterial infection of known aetiology. Follicle formation is the typical response to irritation of all adenoid tissue, and as the conjunctiva contains an adenoid layer it is not surprising that follicles may result from a variety of different irritants. Acute follicular conjunctivitis is a condition in which the palpebral conjunctiva becomes swollen and hyperaemic showing marked follicles, particularly in the upper and lower fornices (Fig. 4). The pre-auricular lymph node is enlarged and the causal agent is probably a virus. The condition improves spontaneously.

Chronic follicular conjunctivitis is a simple hypertrophy of adenoid tissue occurring mainly in children, and although it is probably infective in origin, children with a predisposition to general adenopathy are more likely to be affected.

Vernal conjunctivitis is a bilateral recurrent allergic condition with a seasonal incidence, causing itching and redness of the eyes with lacrimation and some mucous discharge. Young people are more often affected than their elders and the disease appears (in temperate zones) in the early part of the summer and recedes during the autumn and winter. The aetiology is uncertain but is probably an allergic reaction to heat and dust in a sensitive person.

The papules, well illustrated in Fig. 5, occur most commonly on the tarsal conjunctiva but there is a more serious group of cases in which the conjunctiva at the limbus is involved, the lesions spreading onto the cornea which may become completely covered.

17

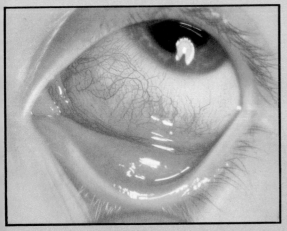

1

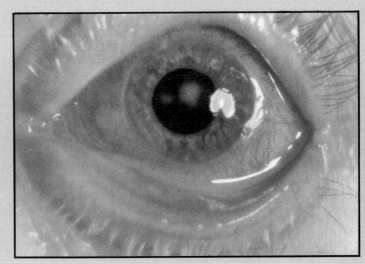

2

FIG. 1.   ACUTE CONJUNCTIVITIS

FIG. 2.   KERATO-CONJUNCTIVITIS

FIG. 3.   TUBERCULOSIS OF THE CONJUNCTIVA

FIG. 4.   FOLLICULAR CONJUNCTIVITIS

FIG. 5.   VERNAL CONJUNCTIVITIS (SPRING CATARRH)

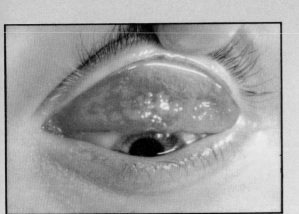

3

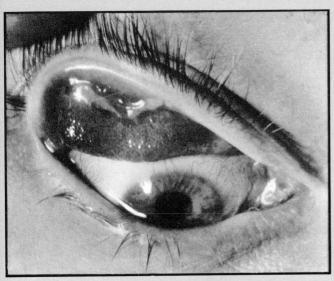

4

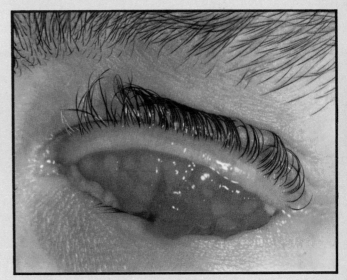

5

Inflammations of the Conjunctiva (cont.)

Phlyctenular conjunctivitis is another type of allergic response by the conjunctiva to an irritant – this time an endogenous agent, typically tuberculo-protein, although other bacterial proteins may have the same effect. It is essentially a disease of children living in overcrowded, unhygienic surroundings on an inadequate diet. Tuberculosis of the lungs or glands is found in a high proportion of cases and enlarged tonsils and adenoids are a common accompaniment.

The phlyctens are raised whitish nodules usually occurring near the limbus and accompanied by a leash of dilated conjunctival vessels (Fig. 1). The nodule tends to ulcerate and finally to disappear, only to be succeeded by a similar lesion at another site. The nodule consists of masses of leucocytes and polymorphonuclear cells in the centre with mononuclear cells and occasional giant cells peripherally.

Sometimes a similar lesion is seen in the cornea where it produces serious disturbance and scarring. Fig. 2 shows such a lesion and its associated leash of blood vessels. The symptoms of phlyctenular conjunctivitis are usually slight but once the cornea is involved pain, lacrimation and photophobia are marked and it may be very difficult to persuade the child to open the lids sufficiently for the eye to be examined.

The treatment is directed to improving the general health by adjusting the diet and living conditions. Sanatorium treatment may be necessary for persistent cases.

Trachoma Although trachoma is a rare disease in England, it is undoubtedly the largest single cause of blindness in the world as a whole. Almost universal in some Middle East countries such as Egypt, it has spread to Asia, India, Central and South America and Africa. It occurs sporadically in southern and eastern Europe.

It is essentially a chronic contagious inflammation of the conjunctiva and cornea with marked sub-epithelial infiltration, follicle formation, vascularization and subsequent scarring. The cicatrization of the palpebral conjunctival lesions of the upper lid causes a severe entropion, the inturned lashes aggravating the already severe corneal lesions.

The aetiological agent is a virus but its identification is still doubtful. Scrapings from the conjunctiva in an active case show numerous inclusion bodies typical of a virus disease, although the exact relationship between the inclusion bodies and the virus is still in doubt. The presence of inclusions, however, is a useful aid to diagnosis.

In the early stages the tarsal conjunctiva shows marked redness with a velvety surface and the cornea shows superficial grey areas. The symptoms are pain, lacrimation and photophobia, largely due to the corneal involvement. The conjunctiva of the upper lids soon becomes hypertrophied and assumes a follicular appearance, while new vessels grow into the cornea from above.

Fig. 3 shows the follicles on the tarsal conjunctiva, and in Fig. 4, the new vessels and diffuse infiltration of the upper half of the cornea can be seen well. Later the follicles become more numerous and may spread into the bulbar conjunctiva. The new vessels and infiltration of the cornea – the trachomatous pannus – progress and are frequently seen in all segments of the cornea, although the upper half is most severely affected. Secondary infection is common. The disease heals through replacement of the follicles by scar formation (Fig. 5) and in the cornea the infiltration becomes less marked but the vessels never completely disappear. If, as is usual, the scarred and contracted upper lid turns inwards, the cornea is damaged by the lashes, a complication which has more serious consequences than the active disease itself.

Recent antibiotic drugs have been found to be very effective in reducing the acute inflammation and preventing secondary infections.

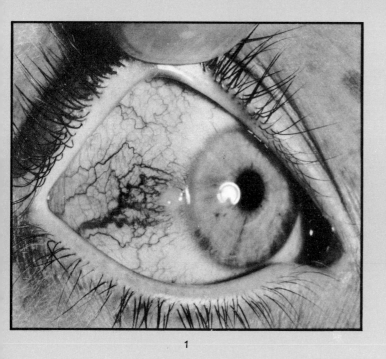

1

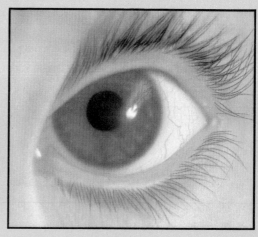

2

FIG. 1. PHLYCTENULAR CONJUNCTIVITIS

FIG. 2. PHLYCTEN OF CORNEA

FIG. 3. TRACHOMA FOLLICLES

FIG. 4. TRACHOMATOUS PANNUS

FIG. 5. TRACHOMATOUS SCARRING OF THE UPPER LID AND CORNEA

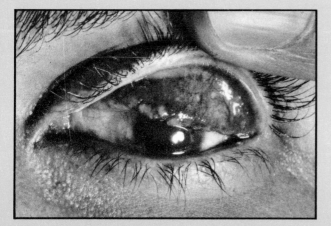

3

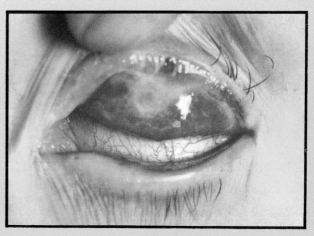

5

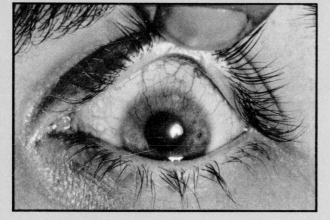

4

Miscellaneous Conjunctival Conditions

Subconjunctival Haemorrhage The sudden appearance of an effusion of blood under the conjunctiva is a common happening in an otherwise normal eye. Sometimes it follows slight trauma or local congestion due to coughing or sneezing but more usually it occurs spontaneously. Vascular diseases such as arteriosclerosis, hypertension and diabetes may be predisposing factors and it may also be seen in purpuric conditions (Fig. 1). Such conditions should, of course, be excluded but in the vast majority of cases a subconjunctival haemorrhage is of no importance. The blood, which is usually in the inter-palpebral portion of the conjunctiva as shown in Fig. 2, is gradually absorbed, changing colour from bright red to yellow. No local treatment is required.

Pinguecula Exposure to wind and dust frequently causes degenerative changes in the inter-palpebral conjunctiva, particularly in older people. The fibrous tissue undergoes hyaline degeneration and the elastic fibres proliferate to form a yellowish nodule, called a pinguecula, on the nasal side of the cornea and later appearing on the lateral side as well (Fig. 3). It is avascular and is frequently unnoticed until an incidental conjunctivitis causes it to stand out clearly against the red background of dilated conjunctival vessels. A pinguecula causes no symptoms and requires no treatment.

Pterygium Although a pterygium is primarily a corneal condition it is included here for comparison with pinguecula. Like the latter condition it is degenerative in nature and is found particularly in people who live in hot dusty climates. Pathologically a pterygium is a degeneration of Bowman's membrane and the superficial corneal lamellae together with replacement by vascularized tissue over which extends the conjunctival epithelium. The process begins at the nasal and temporal borders of the cornea and progresses towards the centre, taking with it a continuation of the conjunctival epithelium (Fig. 4).

In the early stages a pterygium causes no symptoms but when it encroaches on the pupillary region vision is affected. If untreated serious visual disability will result.

Treatment consists in surgical removal and as recurrences are common many different procedures have been devised. Burying the apex beneath healthy conjunctiva is often effective in preventing recurrence.

Pseudo-pterygium is a condition in which conjunctiva becomes adherent to a marginal corneal ulcer and is similarly drawn onto the cornea; it can be distinguished from a true pterygium by the fact that the fold of conjunctiva forms a bridge at the limbus under which a fine probe can be passed.

Argyrosis Silver staining of the conjunctiva may occur as an occupational disease or from the long continued use of drops containing silver nitrate or organic-silver preparations. With the advent of the antibiotic drugs silver preparations are now used much less frequently in ophthalmology and most of the cases seen to-day are due to silver dust from industrial processes. The silver has a particular affinity for the elastic fibres immediately beneath the conjunctival epithelium and in Descemet's membrane. The conjunctiva assumes a dusky hue, particularly marked in the region of the inner canthus, as shown in Fig. 5. Examination with the slit-lamp microscope shows aggregation of the particles along the walls of the conjunctival vessels and a granular deposit in the deeper layers of the substantia propria and Descemet's membrane. The granules of silver cause no irritation or symptoms but the staining is permanent.

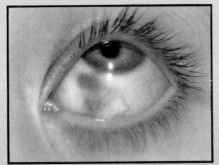

(Guy's Hospital, London)

1

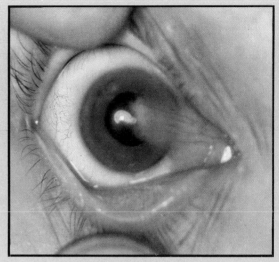

4

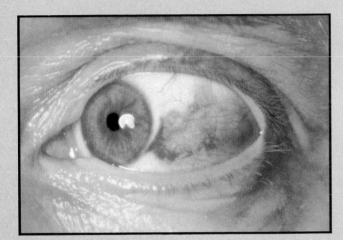

2

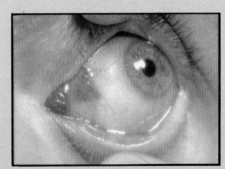

5

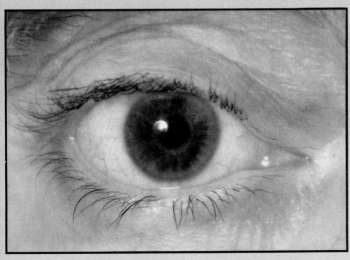

3

FIG. 1.   SUBCONJUNCTIVAL HAEMORRHAGE IN PURPURA

FIG. 2.   ABSORBING CONJUNCTIVAL HAEMORRHAGE

FIG. 3.   PINGUECULAE

FIG. 4.   PTERYGIUM

FIG. 5.   ARGYROSIS

Conjunctival and Epibulbar Tumours

THE CORNEA, being an avascular structure, is very rarely the site of origin of a tumour. Many new growths, however, arise from the limbus, which is the site of transition from conjunctival to corneal epithelium, and these are grouped together under the title of epibulbar tumours.

Epibulbar Dermoid These tumours are present at birth and may be quite small initially, but slowly grow over the cornea. Histologically, they are covered by keratinized stratiform epithelium, often containing hair follicles, underneath which is a miscellaneous collection of elastic fibres, unstriped muscle, blood vessels and nerves. Such a growth is illustrated in Fig. 1. As they tend to increase in size and may cover the pupillary area they are best excised and the remaining scar may be tattooed to render it less obvious.

Haemangioma of the conjunctiva usually takes the form of a cavernous haemangioma consisting of spaces lined with endothelium and containing blood and hyaline debris. The appearance of such a benign tumour is illustrated in Fig. 2; it may arise from conjunctival or from the deeper episcleral vessels. This neoplasm can usually be excised satisfactorily.

Cystic naevus is another type of benign epibulbar tumour which is really congenital in origin although it may not be apparent at birth. It corresponds to a mole of the skin and grows very slowly unless malignant changes supervene. Such tumours are derived from the end-apparatus of sensory nerves and appear as yellowish plaques in the limbal region which, on microscopical examination, are found to consist of groups of large naevus cells in an alveolar formation. Golden granules of melanin are scattered throughout the tumour, being particularly abundant near the surface.

Fig. 3 shows a typical cystic naevus – a yellowish ill-defined tumour with dilated conjunctival vessels supplying it. The cystic nature and pigment granules can be clearly seen with the slit-lamp microscope.

If the tumour is small and does not increase in size it can be left alone, but as the results of malignant change may be disastrous, complete excision should be considered.

Epithelioma occurs typically as an epibulbar tumour but may arise elsewhere in the conjunctiva or at the caruncle. At the limbus the tumour starts as a greyish nodule which extends over the cornea as a fleshy swelling, well illustrated in Fig. 4. The corneal involvement causes a painful keratitis and frequently a secondary iridocyclitis. It tends to grow fairly slowly and does not metastasize to the neighbouring lymph nodes until the later stages, so that the prognosis after enucleation is good.

Sarooma of the conjunctiva is most frequently melanotic in type and may be an epibulbar tumour or may grow from any area of the conjunctiva. The limbal tumours as shown in Fig. 5 are usually more pigmented than the pedunculated type in Fig. 6, which is growing from the palpebral conjunctiva of the upper lid. Histologically they show the typical highly cellular structure of a sarcoma containing many blood vessels. The tumours are very malignant and metastasize early, secondary deposits or orbital recurrences being common in spite of enucleation or even exenteration of the orbit.

23

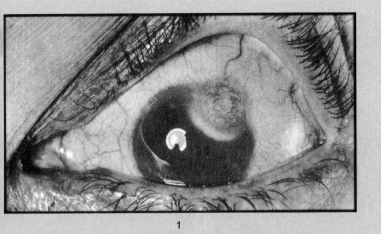

1

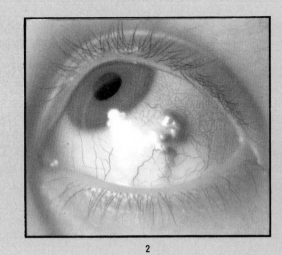

2

FIG. 1.   EPIBULBAR DERMOID

FIG. 2.   CONJUNCTIVAL HAEMANGIOMA

FIG. 3.   CYSTIC NAEVUS OF THE CONJUNCTIVA

FIG. 4.   LIMBAL EPITHELIOMA

FIG. 5.   MELANOTIC SARCOMA OF THE CONJUNCTIVA

FIG. 6.   PEDUNCULATED SARCOMA OF THE CONJUNCTIVA

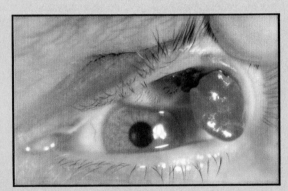

3

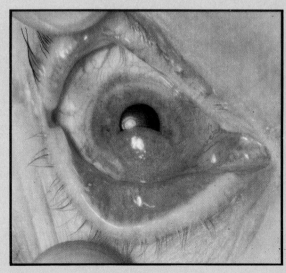

6

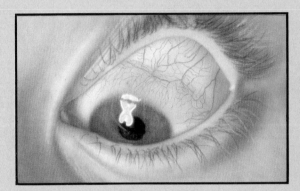

5

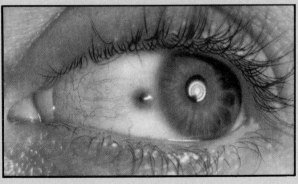

4

Inflammations of the Cornea

INFLAMMATIONS OF THE CORNEA can be divided broadly into superficial ulcerative conditions and deeper (interstitial) inflammations which are usually of endogenous origin.

Dendritic ulcer is a superficial inflammation caused by the virus of herpes simplex. It may follow diseases of the upper respiratory tract or other febrile conditions in the same way as herpes labialis, or it may be a local infection only.

Clinically, the disease starts with an acutely painful eye, with lacrimation and photophobia. The earliest corneal changes consist of fine epithelial opacities with a linear arrangement; these later turn into small vesicles which soon break down leaving raw areas which stain with fluorescein. The pattern produced is of irregular branching lines showing rounded tips to the bifurcations. The corneal sensation is diminished and healing is slow without adequate treatment. Fig. 1 shows the branching pattern of an ulcer which has been stained with fluorescein. The most effective treatment is the application of a strong alcoholic solution of iodine at an early stage combined with atropine and light bandaging.

Hypopyon ulcer starts superficially as a bacterial infection of an epithelial abrasion such as may result from the removal of a corneal foreign body. A hypopyon – a gross exudation of leucocytes and fibrin into the anterior chamber – only accompanies such inflammation when the infective organism is particularly virulent or the patient's resistance is lowered by age or intercurrent disease.

Fig. 2 shows a hazy ulcerated cornea with a definite hypopyon. It is interesting to note that the pupil is contracted – a reflex which may be produced by any irritation of the cornea.

Perforation of the cornea is always to be feared in these severe infections but fortunately Descemet's membrane is very resistant to invasion and intensive antibiotic therapy (by subconjunctival injection) is usually successful in averting such a catastrophe.

Interstitial keratitis may be caused by tuberculosis and other bacterial agents but most cases are syphilitic in origin. It may be a late manifestation of acquired syphilis but it is found most typically in young congenital syphilitics. As a rule the disease is bilateral, although there may be an interval before the second eye is attacked. It starts acutely with pain, lacrimation and photophobia; ciliary injection is marked and the cornea rapidly becomes hazy. Vessels now begin to grow into the cornea to produce the so-called 'salmon-patch', well illustrated in Fig. 3.

The corneal condition is always associated with a uveitis although this is frequently obscured by the opaque cornea. The inflammation continues for two or three months then gradually subsides, leaving a considerable degree of scarring. The vessels which have grown into the cornea never disappear, although in time they cease to carry blood. Such 'ghost' vessels can be seen with the corneal microscope and provide clear evidence of a previous interstitial keratitis. Treatment with penicillin and cortisone reduces the inflammation but must be continued for several months if recurrences are to be avoided.

Rosacea keratitis is a corneal extension of a rosacea conjunctivitis and appears as a marginal infiltration with leashes of superficial vessels crossing the limbus (Fig. 4). It is a chronic condition causing severe disability and pain at the time and permanent loss of vision due to the ensuing corneal scarring.

Local treatment is largely palliative, although corneal grafting may improve the vision considerably when the eye becomes sufficiently quiet for such an operation. There is, however, a marked tendency for the graft to become vascularized and opaque.

Chemical injuries to the cornea are fairly common industrial accidents. Lime burns in particular are frequent and can cause very severe disturbance of the cornea and conjunctiva. Fig. 5 shows the result of a lime burn – a completely opaque cornea with marked ingrowth of blood vessels, an appearance which may be produced by any strong acid or alkali.

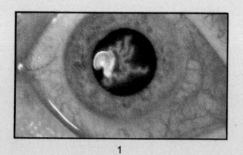

1

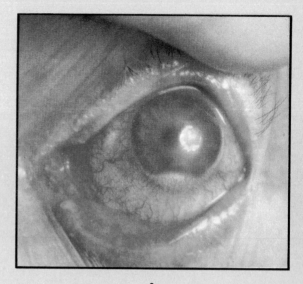

2

FIG. 1. DENDRITIC ULCER

FIG. 2. HYPOPYON ULCER

FIG. 3. INTERSTITIAL KERATITIS

FIG. 4. ROSACEA KERATITIS

FIG. 5. LIME BURN OF THE EYE

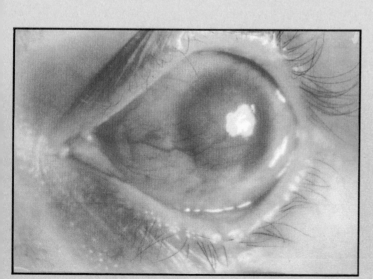

3

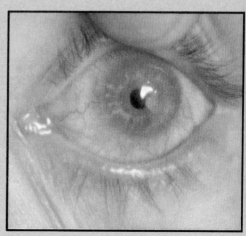

5

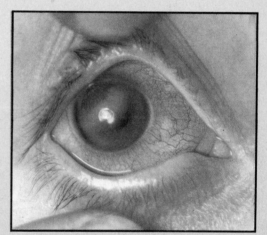

4

Corneal Degenerations

Keratoconus (Conical cornea) This very interesting condition has been included here as a degeneration of the cornea although its true aetiology is still uncertain. It may be developmental and some familial cases have been reported.

Typically the apical bulging of the cornea starts at puberty and increases slowly for several years. The only symptom is deterioration of vision due to the irregular myopic astigmatism caused by the changing corneal curvature. The shape of the cornea is best demonstrated by holding up the upper lid and asking the patient to look down so that the edge of the lower lid follows the corneal curvature across the midline. In the more severe cases the defect is obvious as illustrated in Fig. 1 – a marked case of keratoconus with a normal eye for comparison. In the early stages the vision can be improved by spectacles but soon the refraction becomes too irregular for correction by ordinary lenses. This condition is one in which a most dramatic improvement in vision can be produced by contact lenses. It also responds well to corneal grafting.

Corneal Dystrophies These rare conditions have been described under many different names but can be divided roughly into those affecting primarily the endothelium and epithelium and those affecting the corneal stroma.

It is not uncommon to find some bedewing of the endothelium in elderly patients but this rarely causes any interference with vision. Fuchs's dystrophy, which is illustrated in Fig. 2, starts with a similar endothelial change but progresses to involve the epithelium as well, causing marked oedema and deterioration of vision. The central hazy oedematous area is well shown in Fig. 2.

Many of the stromal dystrophies are familial, the first signs appearing at puberty and slowly progressing throughout life. They are characterized by scattered hyaline changes in the anterior layers of the cornea and the patches may be arranged in many different patterns, lattice-like white lines, rosettes, white rings and other variations.

Fig. 3 is a photograph of a case of Groenouw's corneal dystrophy which has been chosen to illustrate this group of diseases. Whitish spots which may have a ring shape are scattered over the central area of the cornea beneath Bowman's membrane. It is a familial condition and progresses slowly. Corneal grafting offers good hope of visual improvement.

Calcareous Degeneration Calcium salts may be deposited in any site of long-standing hyaline degeneration but are most commonly seen in the cornea following a 'band-shaped degeneration'. In this condition a band of hyaline degeneration stretches across the cornea in the interpalpebral region. Such a case in which calcareous change has developed is illustrated in Fig. 4.

Mooren's Ulcer is a type of degenerative condition found in elderly people which starts as a chronic gutter-like marginal ulcer with undermined edges and may gradually extend across the whole cornea. Such a condition is illustrated in Fig. 5. The aetiology is unknown and the treatment unsatisfactory.

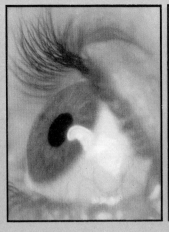
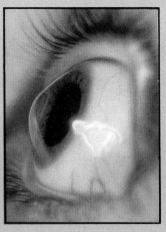

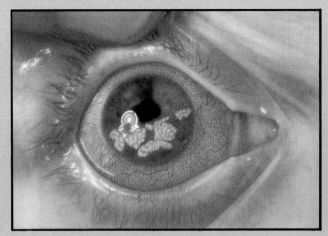

1

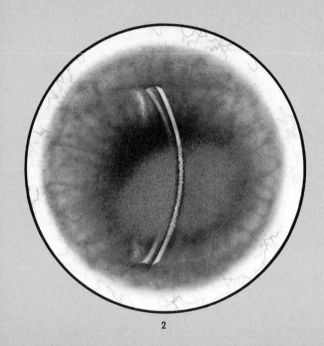

4

FIG. 1. KERATOCONUS (CONICAL CORNEA) COMPARED WITH NORMAL EYE

FIG. 2. FUCHS'S DYSTROPHY

FIG. 3. GROENOUW'S DYSTROPHY

FIG. 4. CALCAREOUS DEGENERATION

FIG. 5. MOOREN'S ULCER

2

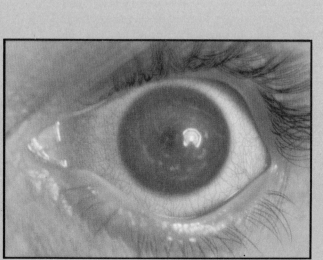

3

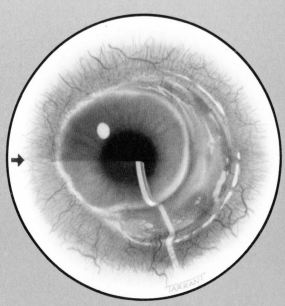

5

Inflammations of the Sclera and Pigmentary Changes

Episcleritis The distinction between an episcleritis in which only the superficial layers of the sclera are involved and a true scleritis is useful clinically, although the pathological process is very similar in the two conditions. Rheumatism and gout have been quoted as common aetiological agents but frequently no cause can be found.

Nodular episcleritis, as its name suggests, is a condition in which raised, localized inflammatory areas arise near the limbus. Fig. 1 shows such a nodule which causes pain and discomfort for some weeks, then disappears, only to recur at another site. The recurrences may continue for several years but the ultimate prognosis is good. Cortisone locally often causes rapid improvement in the condition.

A less severe type of episcleritis occurs in younger people and is characterized by a more diffuse patch of inflammation persisting only for a few hours or days but tending to recur regularly. Symptoms are slight and the condition is probably allergic in nature.

Scleritis Inflammation of the deep layers of the sclera is less common, but much more severe in its manifestations than episcleritis. It may spread forwards to involve the cornea, causing peripheral and even central opacities, and is almost always associated with a severe uveitis.

As shown in Fig. 2, the eye is intensely injected with marked swelling of the subconjunctival tissues. It is a chronic condition accompanied by much pain and diminution of vision. Treatment is unsatisfactory but local and systemic cortisone may be helpful.

Scleromalacia perforans This curious condition is characterized by the appearance of degenerate areas in the sclera which progress to form holes through which uveal tissue tends to prolapse. It is sometimes unaccompanied by any sign of inflammation and occurs in old people with a predisposition to rheumatic disorders.

Fig. 3 shows such a quiet eye in which the darkly pigmented uvea shows under the conjunctiva. Surprisingly enough the condition may exist for many years without causing deterioration of vision.

Melanosis bulbi This is a condition in which the pigment of the uveal tract is greatly increased with the result that the fundus is dark in colour and the iris a deep brown. There is an excess of pigment in the sclera, as shown in Fig. 4 which illustrates the slaty appearance of the sclera below the cornea. The pigment may be in scattered patches or more homogeneously distributed.

Another more serious anomaly of pigmentation which is conjunctival in origin is illustrated in Fig. 5. This condition, called *precancerous melanosis*, is an overgrowth of pigment cells in the conjunctiva and is very liable to develop into a true malignant neoplasm sooner or later. It occurs in adult life and is really a type of intra-epithelial carcinoma.

29

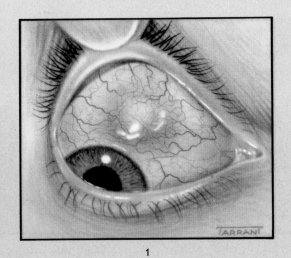

1

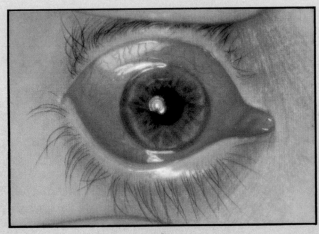

2

FIG. 1. NODULAR EPISCLERITIS

FIG. 2. SCLERITIS

FIG. 3. SCLEROMALACIA PERFORANS

FIG. 4. MELANOSIS BULBI

FIG. 5. PRECANCEROUS MELANOSIS

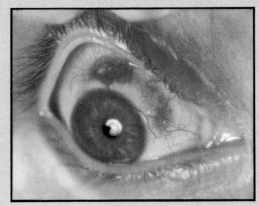

3

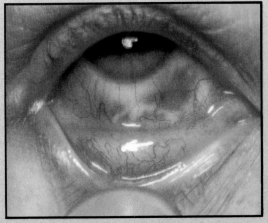

5

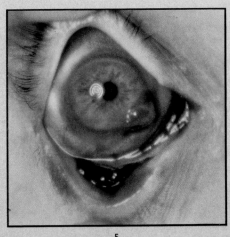

4

Inflammations of the Anterior Uveal Tract

THE UVEAL TRACT comprises the choroid, iris and ciliary body, any part of which may become inflamed, but here the iris and ciliary body only will be discussed.

The general aetiology of uveitis is the same for all parts of the tract. Tuberculosis, sarcoidosis, syphilis and brucellosis are well-known causes, but a large group of cases remains in which no definite aetiological factor can be discovered. These are described as being allergic reactions to an infective agent elsewhere in the body and may be associated with such conditions as ankylosing spondylitis, gout and rheumatism. Clinically, it is possible to group the anterior uveal inflammations broadly into chronic exudative types which show granulomatous nodules (Fig. 1) on the iris and large keratic precipitates (K.P.) on the posterior surface of the cornea, and the more acute or chronic nondescript types with smaller K.P. and no iris nodules. The former group is thought to be caused by actual organismal infection, as by tuberculosis, sarcoidosis, etc., and the latter by an allergic hypersensitivity reaction. Such a classification is almost certainly over-simplified and will undoubtedly be modified when more is known of the aetiology.

Acute Iridocyclitis Pain, photophobia, lacrimation and blurring of vision are the classical symptoms of an acute iridocyclitis. The eye is red, the injection being ciliary in type with a deep flush all round the limbus (Fig. 2). The engorgement of vessels frequently involves those of the iris and, as always in an acute inflammatory process, the hyperaemia is followed by an exudation of protein and cells, in this case into the aqueous of the anterior chamber. The oedema and vascularity of the iris cause a blurring of the iris pattern and the normal coloration becomes less clear. The aqueous humour in a quiet eye is optically empty, which means that if a bright beam of light is thrown across the anterior chamber the aqueous appears dark. When exudate is present, however, some light is reflected back from the protein and cellular elements, giving rise to the so-called 'aqueous flare', in the same way that dust in the air shows in shafts of sunlight. Cells can be seen floating in the beam. Clumps of exudate and cells settle on the posterior surface of the cornea as K.P. – a sure sign of cyclitis – but one which usually requires a loupe or microscope to detect. Fig. 3 is an illustration of K.P. which have been accentuated to show the typical distribution.

Inflammatory irritation of the pupil causes it to constrict, and in the later stages it may become adherent to the anterior surface of the lens (posterior synechiae). Under the influence of a mydriatic the pupil dilates, but when it is partially adherent an irregular shape results, as is seen in Fig. 4.

The iris and ciliary body are always involved together in inflammatory processes, but sometimes the cyclitic element predominates. In these cases there is minimal injection, little change in the iris, but marked K.P. Exudate may also form membranes over the lens and the lens itself may become opaque, a cataract developing, as is shown in Fig. 5.

The plasmoid aqueous of an acute iridocyclitis drains less easily from the anterior chamber and the ocular tension may rise. If the pupil becomes occluded or completely adherent to the lens, a severe secondary glaucoma may ensue.

31

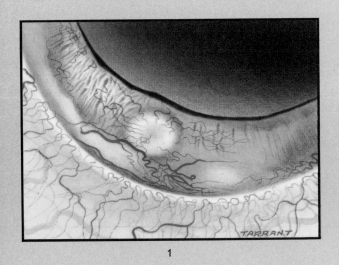

1

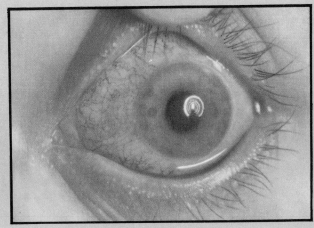

2

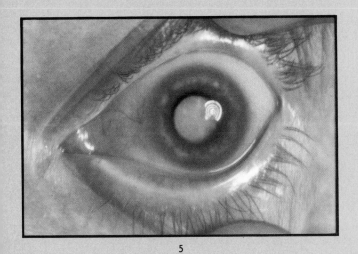

3

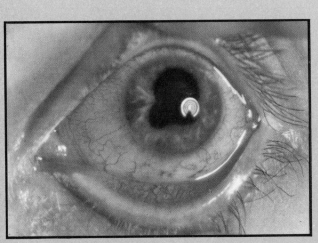

4

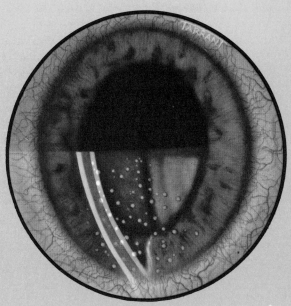

5

FIG. 1. TUBERCULOUS IRITIS

FIG. 2. ACUTE IRIDOCYCLITIS

FIG. 3. K.P. (KERATIC PRECIPITATES)

FIG. 4. POSTERIOR SYNECHIAE

FIG. 5. CATARACT SECONDARY TO IRIDOCYCLITIS

Trauma to the Anterior Segment

Perforating Wounds of the cornea frequently involve the iris and lens. The pupil constricts in response to injury, and as the aqueous leaks out of the corneal wound the iris tends to prolapse through the opening. If the wound is small, the prolapse acts as a plug and allows the anterior chamber to re-form. Such an injury is illustrated in Fig. 1, in which the knuckle of prolapsed iris shows as a dark blob at the site of perforation of the cornea – in this case near the limbus at seven o'clock. If the patient is seen within a few hours and the nature of the perforating object is such that infection is unlikely, it is sometimes justifiable to replace the prolapse and suture the corneal wound. Usually, however, it is safer to excise the prolapse rather than risk replacing infected tissue inside the eye.

Iridodialysis The thinnest part of the iris is at its origin from the ciliary body, and a contusion of the eye may tear the iris at this point, causing an iridodialysis. Such an injury is illustrated in Fig. 2, in which the iris can be seen detached from the ciliary body in two arcs over the lower segment. The pupil is flattened in the region of the dialysis.

Dislocation of the Lens Contusion injuries may rupture the zonule of the lens and cause its dislocation. Usually the lens is displaced laterally or downwards, as in Fig. 3, where the edge of the opaque cataractous lens shows clearly in the pupillary area. This illustration also shows a hypertrophy of black iris pigment over the front surface of the iris. More rarely the lens is dislocated forwards into the anterior chamber, where it is very liable to block the drainage of aqueous and cause a secondary glaucoma. Fig. 4 is a painting of an opaque lens dislocated into the anterior chamber, and the accompanying diagram shows the relative position of the iris and lens.

Foreign Bodies in the Eye A wide variety of foreign bodies may enter the eye in injuries. The commonest are small fragments of metal from hammer-and-chisel accidents or from moving parts of machinery. It must be emphasized that the immediate symptoms of this type of injury may be slight and a small corneal wound is easily overlooked. Radiographs of the eye should be taken after every injury in which it is at all possible that a foreign body may have entered the eye, as any small fragment which has perforated the globe will almost certainly be metallic. Glass may not be revealed by radiography, but usually the history will suggest the possibility of its presence, and examination with a slit-lamp microscope may enable it to be seen in the anterior segment.

Fig. 5 is an illustration of a small metallic foreign body which has entered the anterior chamber through the cornea.

33

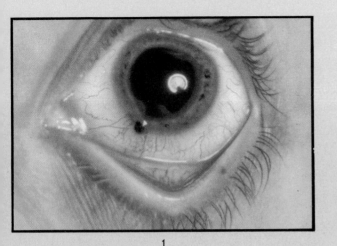

1

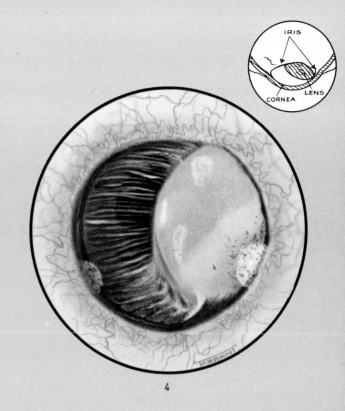

4

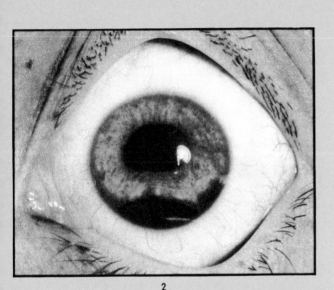

2

FIG. 1.   PERFORATING WOUND WITH PROLAPSED IRIS

FIG. 2.   IRIDODIALYSIS

FIG. 3.   DISLOCATION OF LENS

FIG. 4.   ANTERIOR DISLOCATION OF LENS

FIG. 5.   FOREIGN BODY IN ANTERIOR CHAMBER

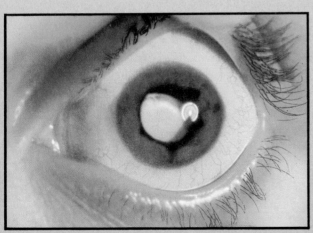

3

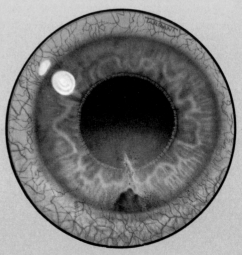

5

Neoplasms of the Anterior Uveal Tract

THE LENS, being an avascular structure, is never the site of a new growth, but the iris and ciliary body may be the site of tumours similar to those occurring in the choroid, the commonest being neuro-ectodermal in origin.

Naevus Small accumulations of pigment are very common in the iris and are usually of no importance. The larger naevi, as illustrated in Fig. 1, may, however, grow and undergo malignant change. Rarely, they are highly vascular (Fig. 2), and may bleed into the anterior chamber, causing a hyphaema. Naevi of the ciliary body cannot be seen clinically but have been seen histologically in eyes sectioned for other reasons.

Malignant Melanoma of the Iris is a rare disease, and the majority of those reported have arisen from a pre-existing naevus. The latter may appear unchanged for many years and then quite suddenly increase in size and become more vascular. The infiltration of the iris reduces its mobility and causes distortion of the pupil, which can be clearly seen in Figs 3 and 4. The growth spreads to the ciliary body and tends to block the angle of the anterior chamber, causing glaucoma. In the early stages it may be possible to excise the portion of iris containing the tumour, but if not the eye must be enucleated.

Leiomyoma of the Iris is a tumour characterized histologically by closely-packed bundles of long, spindle-shaped cells resembling a melanoma but arising from the muscle of the iris. Clinically, it is impossible to distinguish from a melanoma. It is a lightly pigmented yellowish tumour which grows slowly and is relatively benign. Fig. 5 is a photograph of such a tumour, which half fills the anterior chamber. Metastases do not occur, but the neoplasm may recur locally if not completely removed.

Malignant melanoma of the ciliary body is usually unnoticed until it extends forwards as a pigmented mass at the base of the iris or unless lens changes occur causing visual deterioration. The tumour can usually be seen through the fully dilated pupil. Malignant melanomata of the ciliary body tend to infiltrate the sclera, and may be seen emerging under the conjunctiva at the limbus. Fig. 6 shows a malignant melanoma of the choroid and ciliary body which has extended forwards over the base of the iris and outwards through the sclera.

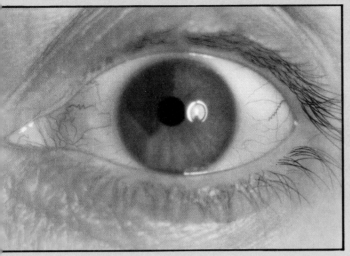

1

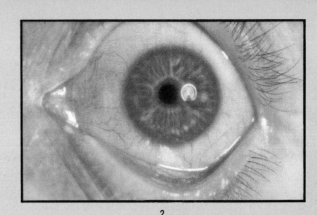

2

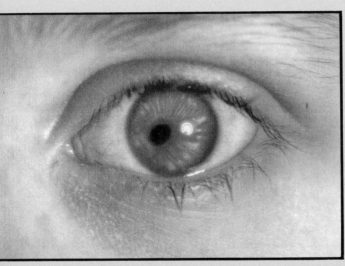

3

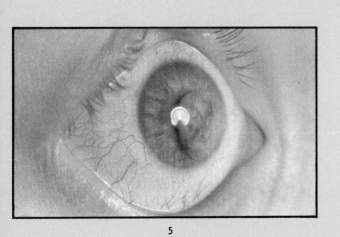

4

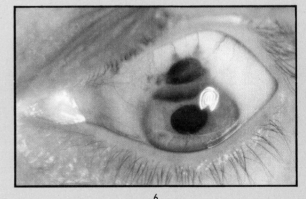

5

6

FIG. 1.   PIGMENTED NAEVUS OF IRIS

FIG. 2.   VASCULAR NAEVUS OF IRIS

FIG. 3.   DISTORTION OF PUPIL BY MALIGNANT MELANOMA

FIG. 4.   ENLARGED VIEW OF MALIGNANT MELANOMA OF IRIS

FIG. 5.   LEIOMYOMA OF IRIS

FIG. 6.   INFILTRATING MELANOMA OF CHOROID

The Lens

Congenital Cataract It will be remembered that the lens is ectodermal in origin and that new fibres are formed by the elongation of the epithelial cells at the equator. Thus, as more lens fibres are laid down, the earlier fibres become centrally placed. Any injury or disturbance of metabolism may render opaque the fibres which are being formed at that time, and therefore the position of the opacity in the lens gives an accurate date to the incident. New fibres continue to be formed throughout life, but very much more slowly than in the foetus.

Congenital lens opacities of many varieties have been recognized and described since the early days of ophthalmology but remained pathological curiosities until the work of Gregg opened up new horizons in their aetiology and, indeed, that of many other congenital defects. In 1941, Gregg noticed that following an epidemic of rubella many of the children whose mothers had contracted the disease in the first two months of pregnancy were born with cataract, sometimes associated with congenital heart disease.

Unless the lens is completely opaque congenital cataracts may not be noticed until the child is found to have a visual defect.

Fig. 1 illustrates a zonular cataract, one of the many types of congenital lens changes. Some of the fibres laid down during development are abnormal and form a partially opaque zone between the embryonic nucleus and the cortex of the lens. Such congenital cataracts are usually bilateral and surgical treatment is indicated if the reduction in visual acuity is sufficient to hinder normal development.

Small punctate bluish opacities are a common finding in normal eyes, and represent occasional lens fibres which have not developed normally. If such opacities are marked, they are known as blue-dot cataracts (Fig. 2). Vision is rarely affected.

Coronary Cataract is a type of developmental cataract appearing soon after puberty. Numerous club-shaped whitish opacities can be seen in the peripheral cortex of the lens, often associated with 'blue-dot' changes (Fig. 3). Such appearances can be found in many people, but as they are peripheral and of very slow progression, rarely produce any visual defect.

Ectopia Lentis If the suspensory ligament of the lens is absent or weakened over a segment, the whole lens becomes displaced away from the weak portion. Such displacement is called ectopia lentis and occurs not uncommonly as a congenital and often hereditary defect (Fig. 4). When the pupil is well dilated, it is possible to see the fundus ophthalmoscopically through the lens and also round the edge of the lens.

Ectopia lentis may be a component of a widespread mesodermal defect known as Marfan's syndrome, characterized by an elongation of the long bones, particularly of the hands and feet, undeveloped musculature and infantilism. The long, spidery fingers have given the disease the name of arachnodactyly. Fig. 5 is a photograph of the hand of a six-year-old boy with this condition. The ectopia is often associated with myopia and astigmatism, and the weakened zonule predisposes to traumatic dislocation of the lens.

37

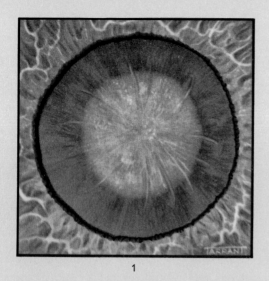

1

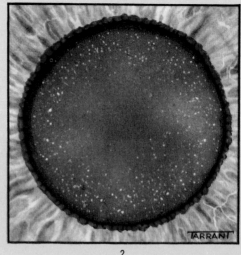

2

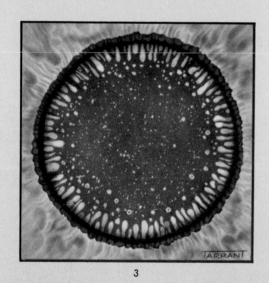

3

FIG. 1.   ZONULAR CATARACT

FIG. 2.   'BLUE-DOT' CATARACT

FIG. 3.   CORONARY CATARACT

FIG. 4.   ECTOPIA LENTIS

FIG. 5.   ARACHNODACTYLY

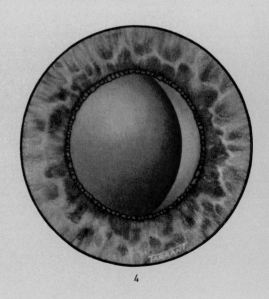

5

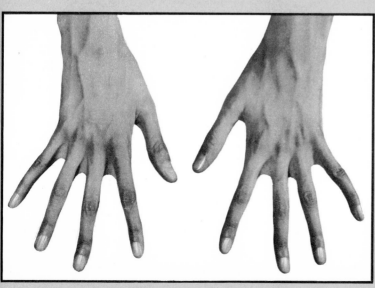

4

The Lens (cont.)

Senile Cataract Some degree of lenticular sclerosis is always present in old age and can be recognized by the increased scattering of light from the lens. This is evidenced by the slightly greyish appearance of the pupil in old people compared to the jet black pupil of young people. The effect on vision, however, is insignificant, and usually no opacity will be seen with the ophthalmoscope.

Senile cataract usually commences in the peripheral cortical areas and can be seen with a +12 D lens in the ophthalmoscope as dark spokes at the periphery of the lens against the red reflex from the fundus. Fig. 1 is a photograph of a typical senile cataract in which the peripheral spokes and opacities are silhouetted against reflected light from the fundus. Nuclear sclerosis will produce much more serious interference with vision and will require operative treatment earlier than the more usual peripheral opacities.

With modern operative technique it is no longer necessary to wait for a cataract to become 'ripe' (*i.e.* complete opacification of the lens) before it can be extracted, and the criterion for operation now is the visual disability of the patient.

Diabetic Cataract Although it is common to find senile lens changes at an earlier age in diabetics than in other patients, a true diabetic cataract is rare. When it does occur, it is usually in a young person and often progresses very rapidly, the lens becoming completely opaque in a matter of weeks. The opacity is in the superficial layers of the cortex and consists of numerous white spots and fluid vacuoles, as shown in the slit-lamp drawing (Fig. 2).

Complicated Cataract Any severe disease of the inner eye, such as a long-standing uveitis, detached retina or intra-ocular neoplasm, may derange the metabolic processes of the lens sufficiently to cause cataract. Chronic uveitis is the most common offender; Fig. 3 shows an eye with uveitis and a mature cataract. The upper part of the iris has been removed surgically, but elsewhere it has an atrophic appearance and is adherent to the lens by numerous posterior synechiae. The changes start at the posterior pole and often show a typical polychromatic lustre when seen with the slit-lamp microscope. Fig. 4 shows posterior cortical changes in the lens complicating a tuberculous uveitis, as seen by direct illumination and with the ophthalmoscope.

Dermatogenous Cataract As the lens is an ectodermal tissue, it is not surprising to find cataract associated with some skin diseases. Neurodermatitis, scleroderma, poikiloderma and chronic eczema may all be associated with cataractous changes. Fig. 5 is an illustration of those occurring in a case of Besnier's prurigo. The opacity forms a bluish plaque in the anterior cortical region.

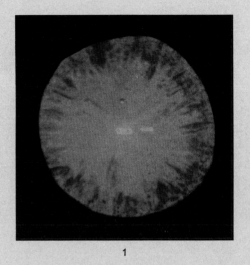

1

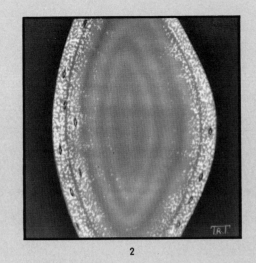

2

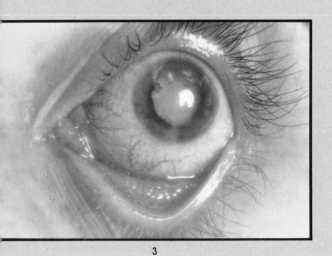

3

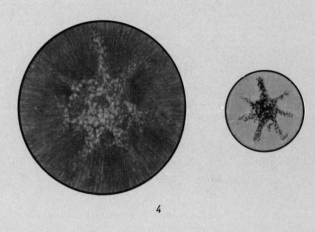

4

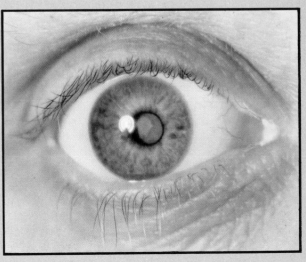

5

FIG. 1.   PHOTOGRAPH OF SENILE CATARACT

FIG. 2.   DIABETIC CATARACT

FIG. 3.   COMPLICATED CATARACT

FIG. 4.   POSTERIOR CORTICAL LENS CHANGES

        (*Left*) BY DIRECT ILLUMINATION

        (*Right*) OPHTHALMOSCOPICALLY

FIG. 5.   CATARACT ACCOMPANYING BESNIER'S PRURIGO

Gonioscopy

THE ANGLE OF THE ANTERIOR CHAMBER is of particular importance in the study of glaucoma but is normally hidden from direct view by the overlapping of the sclera at the limbus. If, however, the refraction of the cornea is cancelled by the application of a suitable contact lens, it is possible to view the angle microscopically. The contact lens may be dome-shaped, as in the Koeppe and Barkan designs, or conical with a mirror to reflect an image of the angle forwards, as in the Goldmann type, the optical principles of which are illustrated in Fig. 1. The dome-shaped lenses are designed for use with a hand-held binocular loupe or microscope, while the Goldmann lens is for use with the slit-lamp microscope.

Fig. 2 shows diagrammatically the structures to be seen in a normal broad angle. Beyond the last folds of the iris can be seen the base of the ciliary body. The red line indicates the position of the canal of Schlemm, which shows up most clearly when filled with blood. This is not the normal state of affairs but can often be produced by pressure on the globe. Above the canal of Schlemm can be seen Schwalbe's line, which marks the end of the trabeculae. It is through this lattice-like structure that the aqueous humour drains to reach the canal of Schlemm and find an exit from the eye; this structure is also shown in section in the illustration.

Fig. 3 shows in similar diagrammatic form the appearance of a narrow angle. Here the deeper recesses of the angle are hidden by the iris and only Schwalbe's line can be seen.

Congestive glaucoma is associated with a shallow anterior chamber and a narrow angle, and it is easy to see from the above diagram that dilatation of the pupil would cause a bunching-up of the iris thus blocking the drainage of aqueous from the anterior chamber. In chronic simple glaucoma the anterior chamber is of average depth and the angle is not narrowed.

In glaucoma secondary to iridocyclitis the angle is usually found to be partly or completely blocked by exudates and adhesions between the root of the iris and the cornea (anterior peripheral synechiae).

Apart from its use in glaucoma, gonioscopy is also valuable in assessing the extent of neoplasms of the iris and ciliary body, and for the detection of foreign bodies in the angle.

Fig. 4 shows the gonioscopic appearance of the interesting but rare condition of *aniridia*. This congenital defect implies a complete absence of the iris, but it can be seen from this illustration that there is still a small fringe of iris present on the anterior surface of the ciliary body. The ciliary processes, the zonule of the lens and the border of the lens itself can be clearly seen. The whitish tissue above the stump of the iris is anomalous tissue covering the trabeculae, causing an embarrassment of the normal drainage channels, which may result in glaucoma.

41

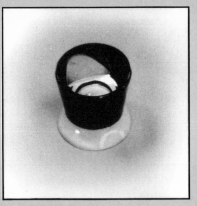

1a

A. Schwalbe's line

B. Position of canal of Schlemm

C. Trabeculae

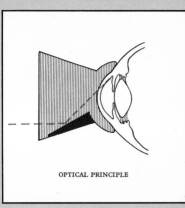

OPTICAL PRINCIPLE

1b

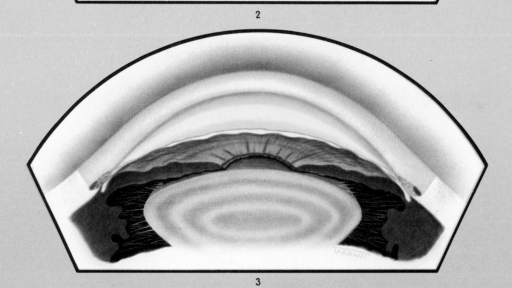

2

3

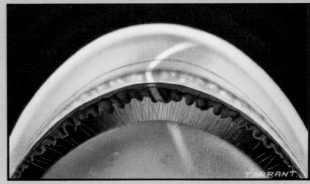

4

FIG. 1, a & b. GOLDMANN CONTACT LENS AND OPTICAL PRINCIPLE

FIG. 2.   NORMAL BROAD ANGLE

FIG. 3.   NORMAL NARROW ANGLE

FIG. 4.   ANIRIDIA AS SEEN WITH THE GONIOSCOPE

Miscellaneous Conditions of the Uveal Tract and Lens

Heterochromic Cyclitis   This is a disease of young adults in which a quiet cyclitis with precipitates on the back of the cornea is accompanied by an atrophy of the iris tissue, causing it to appear much paler than the fellow eye, and the development of lens changes. The aetiology of the condition is obscure. Fig. 1 shows well the paler iris of the affected eye.

Coloboma of the Iris   Incomplete fusion of the optic cup results in colobomatous defects in the uveal tract. Mild degrees of coloboma of the iris are quite common and appear as a deficiency of iris stroma, usually situated at six o'clock, allowing the pigment epithelium to show more clearly as a dark spot.

Fig. 2 is a photograph of a patient with a complete cleft in the lower part of the iris which can be clearly seen against the background of an opaque lens. Coloboma of the choroid may be associated with such defects.

Cysts in the Anterior Chamber and Iris   The two commonest types of cyst formation in the anterior chamber and iris are congenital and traumatic implantation cysts. It is probable that the congenital type is due to an epithelial out-pouching into the underlying mesoderm in a manner similar to the formation of the lens vesicle. Fig. 3 is an illustration of such a cyst seen with the slit-lamp microscope. The implantation cysts are due to the introduction of small pieces of corneal or conjunctival epithelium into the anterior chamber by a perforating injury or at operation.

Senile Exfoliation of the Lens Capsule   This condition is illustrated in Fig. 4 by a case in which a glaucoma iridectomy has been performed. Fine white flakes, which are now considered to be a deposit from the aqueous and not a true exfoliation of lens capsule, can be seen adhering to the margin of the pupil and to the centre and periphery of the anterior surface of the lens. Gonioscopy shows similar deposits in the angle of the anterior chamber where they cause an obstruction to the outflow of aqueous with the development of glaucoma in a high proportion (up to 70 per cent) of all cases.

Retrolental Fibroplasia

RETROLENTAL FIBROPLASIA is the name given to a vascular hyperplasia of the peripheral retina which forms a membrane behind the lens. The natural history of the disease is most interesting. It was first described in 1942, and over the next few years assumed such proportions that it ranked as a major cause of blindness in children in the U.S.A. and in Britain. It was soon realized that the condition rarely occurred except in premature infants, and several theories as to its aetiology were advanced. Experimental researches and careful clinical controls have now established that almost all cases are due to an excessive use of oxygen. It has been shown in kittens that high concentrations of oxygen can cause a complete obliteration of the growing retinal vessels. On transfer to air the obliterated vessels only partially reopen, so that a severe anoxia occurs within the retinal tissue. This provokes a profuse formation of new vessels with glomerular tufts and loops extending into the vitreous, giving a histological picture very similar to that seen in the early stages of retrolental fibroplasia. In infants the neovascularization is followed by retinal detachment, and it is this detached tissue which produces the typical appearance of a vascularized sheet behind the lens (Figs 5 and 6).

43

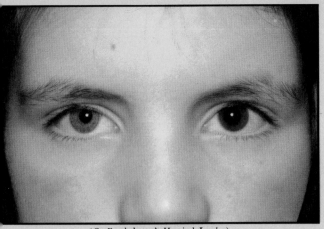

(*St. Bartholomew's Hospital, London*)

1

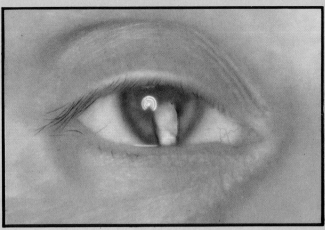

2

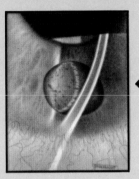

3

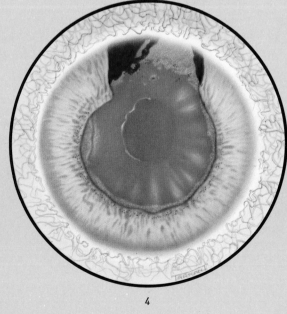

5

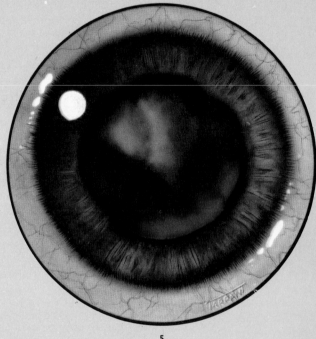

4

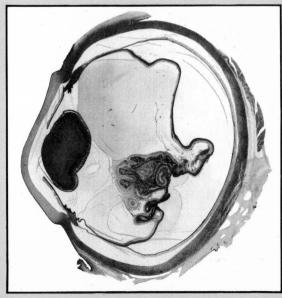

6

FIG. 1.   HETEROCHROMIA OF IRIS

FIG. 2.   COLOBOMA OF IRIS

FIG. 3.   CYST IN ANTERIOR CHAMBER

FIG. 4.   SENILE EXFOLIATION OF LENS CAPSULE

FIG. 5.   RETROLENTAL FIBROPLASIA

FIG. 6.   SECTION OF EYE WITH RETROLENTAL FIBROPLASIA

The Normal Fundus

SEEN OPHTHALMOSCOPICALLY, the normal fundus varies within wide limits. What may be described as two very typical examples are seen in Figs 1 and 2, the first as taken by the fundus camera ($\times 2 \times 5 = \times 10$), and the second as seen with the ophthalmoscope ($\times 12$) and depicted by an artist; the comparison afforded by these two techniques will frequently be used in the following sections. The most prominent feature is the optic disc, round or slightly oval in shape, which marks the entrance of the optic nerve. Situated centrally in Fig. 2, it stands out sharply, paler than the general aspect of the fundus and normally has a well-defined margin. It dips down slightly in the centre into a physiological cup which varies considerably in depth and configuration in different eyes, and from it the retinal vessels radiate, dividing dichotomously into innumerable branches as they spread over the fundus. Their walls are normally transparent and the blood column in the arteries appears a brighter red than the slightly purplish veins. Moreover, the arteries are narrower and show a slightly more brilliant bright streak than the veins, because the light is reflected partly from the convex cylindrical blood column and partly from the media of the walls.

The Macula is the most important region of the fundus, since it subserves central vision. It lies some two disc diameters to the temporal side of the optic disc and somewhat below its centre. It is depicted in Fig. 3. It is usually slightly deeper in tint than the surrounding fundus, owing to the greater thickness of the subjacent choriocapillaris. In its centre is a small pit, the fovea, which normally appears as a bright reflex, since the light of the ophthalmoscope is reflected from its curved walls. The reflex varies considerably in shape and intensity, but the illustration shows one of the more simple and common appearances.

General Pigmentation of the background of the fundus varies between individuals. If the pigment is deficient, the choroidal vessels may sometimes be seen; they are distinguished from the retinal vessels in that they have no central reflex, are broader and anastomose freely. In heavily pigmented people the fundus is a darker red, and if the retinal epithelium preponderates it shows a fine pigmented stippling, while if the choroidal pigment is dense in comparison with that of the retinal epithelium, the polygonal areas between the choroidal vessels appear darkly outlined, giving the appearance of a *tesselated* or *tigroid* fundus, seen in Fig. 6. In dark races the whole fundus is of a somewhat darker colour; the typical fundus of a native of Africa is seen in Fig. 4. Among the yellow races a dark or even slate colour is more pronounced, as is seen in Fig. 5, which is the typical fundus of a native of China. A tracery of light-reflexes is seen emanating from the disc following the course of the nerve fibres running therefrom out into the fundus; this is a non-pathological appearance seen by the ophthalmoscope in fundi of all types.

45

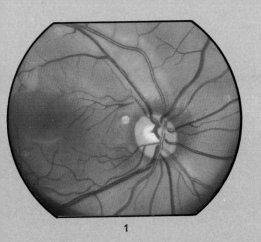

1

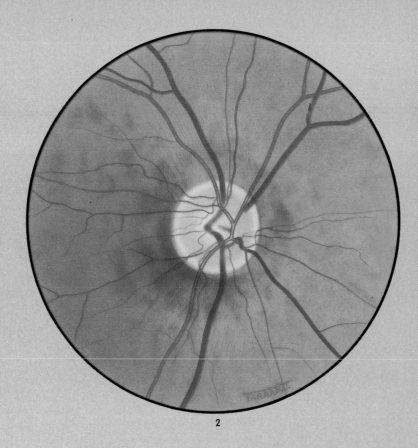

2

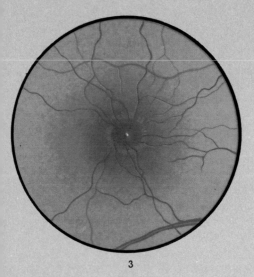

3

FIG. 1. FUNDUS PHOTOGRAPH (MAGNIFICATION × 10).

FIG. 2. FUNDUS PAINTING (MAGNIFICATION × 12)

FIG. 3. THE MACULAR REGION

FIG. 4. FUNDUS OF AN AFRICAN NATIVE

FIG. 5. FUNDUS OF AN ASIATIC

FIG. 6. TIGROID FUNDUS

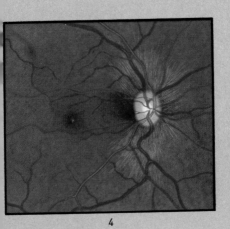

4

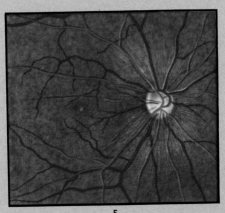

5

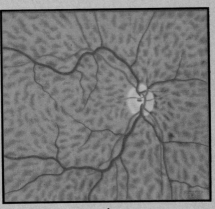

6

Arteriosclerosis

A DIFFUSE DEGENERATION of the media is an almost universal finding in the arteries of older patients, but the recognition of such changes in the retinal vessels is complicated by the hypertensive changes that so frequently accompany arteriosclerosis.

In the absence of hypertension the earliest changes are an increase in light reflex from the arterial wall and masking of the veins at the arterio-venous crossings. Normally it is possible to distinguish a vein through the overlying artery, but when the arterial wall becomes thickened, this is no longer possible. Later the arteries become more tortuous and show irregularities of calibre, well seen in Fig. 1. The irregularity is most marked near the disc and frequently the blood stream is narrowed to a fine thread for a section of the vessel.

At the arterio-venous crossings the veins become nipped and deflected so as to meet the arteries more nearly at a right angle, and the peripheral section of the vein becomes engorged.

Vascular Occlusion The constriction of the vein may be sufficient to cause thrombotic occlusion, and in Fig. 2 such an accident has occurred at the first crossing of the superior temporal artery and vein. A collateral circulation has developed, the new channel now lying over the artery instead of beneath it. The appearance of new vessel formation in an arteriosclerotic retina is pathognomonic of a vascular occlusion. The central artery or any branch of it may also become occluded, with serious visual consequences.

Advanced Appearances The arteries assume a 'copper wire' appearance due to increased reflection of light from the vessel wall and in the later stages small haemorrhages and hard white exudates develop, particularly in the macular region. This is well shown in Fig. 3.

The exudates are in marked contrast to the paler fluffy patches seen in the more acute hypertensive retinopathy. The sclerosis of the arterial wall may proceed to such a degree that the blood column cannot be seen at all and the vessels appear as bright streaks – so-called 'silver wiring', but such extreme sclerosis is almost always accompanied by some degree of hypertension. Increased density of the arterial wall may also be shown by sheathing of the vessels, as in Fig. 1.

Retinal oedema is a characteristic of hypertensive retinopathy, and is never found as a result of purely arteriosclerotic changes, otherwise the difference between the fundus appearances in arteriosclerosis and hypertension is largely one of degree, the arteriosclerotic changes merging imperceptibly into the hypertensive as the blood-pressure rises.

Purely arteriosclerotic vascular changes in the retina may be unaccompanied by any visual symptoms. It is only when the macula shows signs of degeneration or an artery or vein becomes occluded that vision is affected.

The macular lesions tend to become slowly but steadily worse. Venous occlusion of a branch of the central vein causes a quadrantic type of field loss corresponding to the area of retina drained by the vein and some disturbance of macular vision is the rule if either temporal branch is affected. In these cases some improvement in central vision is to be expected when the oedema and haemorrhages are absorbed.

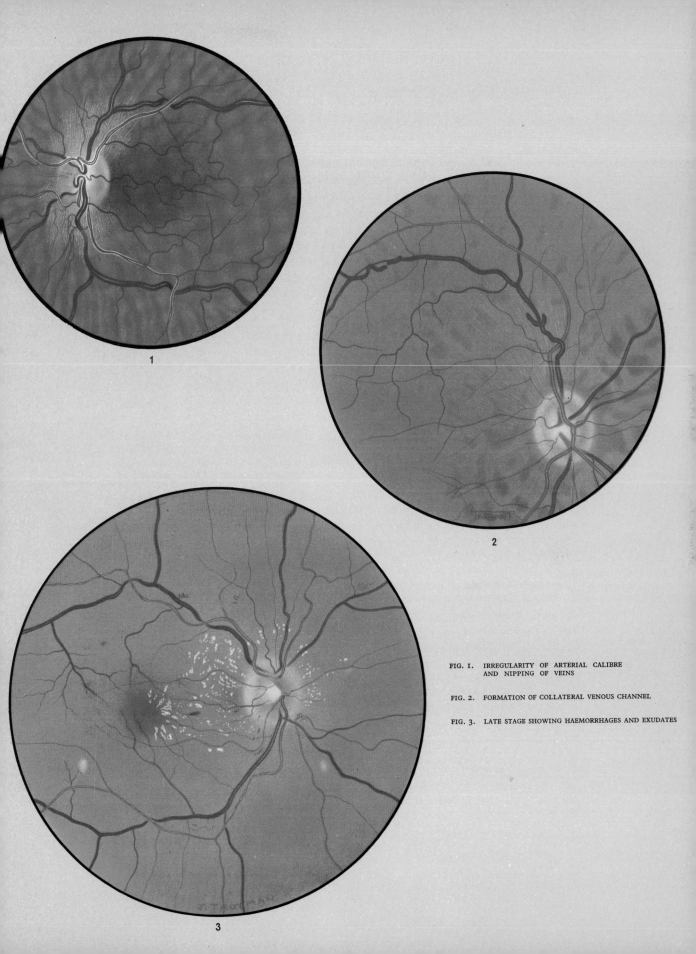

FIG. I. IRREGULARITY OF ARTERIAL CALIBRE
AND NIPPING OF VEINS

FIG. 2. FORMATION OF COLLATERAL VENOUS CHANNEL

FIG. 3. LATE STAGE SHOWING HAEMORRHAGES AND EXUDATES

The Fundus in Hypertension

THE PICTURE of hypertensive retinopathy is one of the most dramatic in ophthalmology and is also of unusual importance from the point of view of general medicine, since it provides a clear and unequivocal view of the state of the arterioles and reflects particularly the condition of the vessels of corresponding size in the cerebral circulation. A knowledge of the more common appearances is therefore of great importance to the physician as well as to the ophthalmologist. The picture, of course, is frequently complicated by secondary effects due to renal damage, so that the characteristics of a hypertensive and a renal retinopathy may well be combined. The common changes include alterations in the retinal blood vessels and more widespread results of oedema and exudation into the retinal tissues.

The Arteries   Sometimes the retinal changes appear acutely in a relatively normal fundus, especially in young persons, but usually they are associated with the narrow, attenuated arteries characteristic of hypertension of some duration. This is particularly well seen in Fig. 5. The arterial constriction may be preceded by evidences of angiospasm and may progress to partial or complete obliteration of the arteries, a phenomenon well seen in the vessels running upwards and outwards above the macula in Fig. 6. In this illustration two of the arteries appear as solid white strands. The dense, hard arteries quite frequently press on, and may almost obliterate, the veins as they cross over them, a phenomenon clearly seen in the inferior artery in Fig. 1. The changes in the eye even in advanced cases may be confined to these alterations in the arteries, but in most cases of long-standing further pathological evidences appear. One of these is the appearance of miliary aneurysms due to degenerative changes in the walls of the blood vessels. A fairly large aneurysm and a cluster of small ones are seen in the horizontal meridian of Fig. 6, towards the left. The more common appearance, however, is that of haemorrhages, sometimes small and flame-shaped, lying in the more superficial layers of the retina, at other times round and more deeply located; both types are well seen in Figs 1 and 4.

Oedema   One of the characteristics of the fundus in hypertension is the presence of oedema, which may be massive. An early stage is seen in Fig. 4, where the swelling of the retinal tissues has produced light reflexes radiating out from the disc. In Fig. 5 the oedema has been more pronounced and the entire disc is fuzzy; in a more advanced stage still the picture of papilloedema, almost indistinguishable from that presented by a cerebral tumour, may be present.

Exudates   The patches of exudate may be large and extremely numerous. They may pepper the fundus, appearing as soft-contoured 'woolly' masses, such as are seen round the disc in Fig. 4. These may harden and become smaller, more discrete and sharply delineated, as in Fig. 2 and in the macular region of Fig. 4; while they may pile themselves up in heaps to form an extensive peripapillary ring, as in Fig. 3, widely diffused sheets or a macular star, as in Fig. 5. The presence of exudates is indicative of renal involvement of some severity, and in such cases the prognosis in general is not good.

49

FIG. I.   OBLITERATION OF VEINS AT ARTERIO-VENOUS CROSSINGS

FIG. 2.   OLD EXUDATES ROUND THE DISC

FIG. 3.   EXTENSIVE PERIPAPILLARY EXUDATES

FIG. 4.   'WOOLLY' EXUDATES

FIG. 5.   'STAR' FIGURE AT MACULA

FIG. 6.   ANEURYSM FORMATION

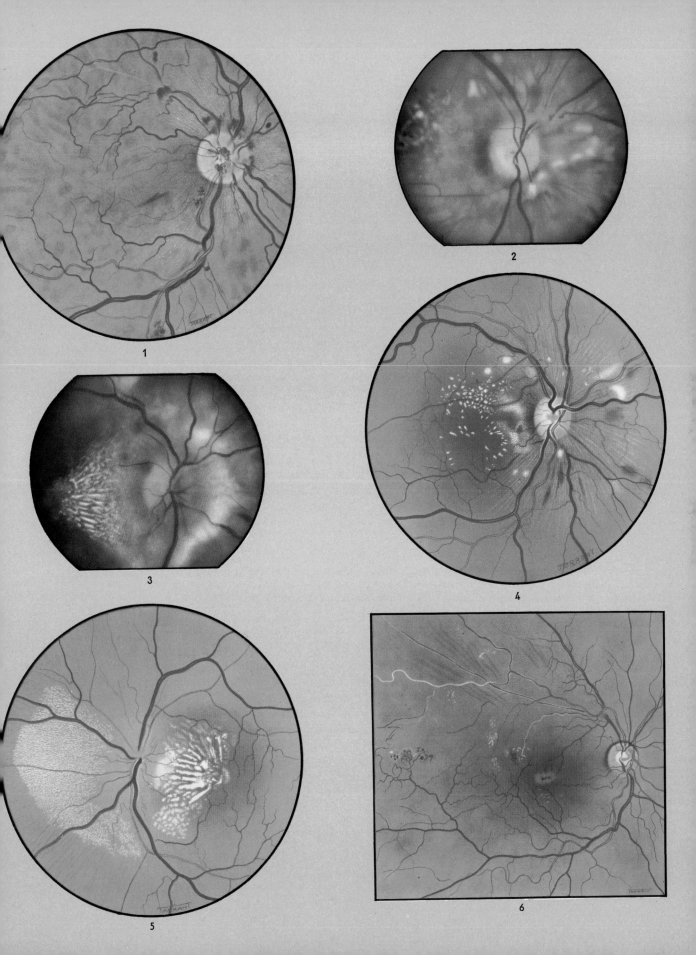

1

2

3

4

5

6

Diabetic Retinopathy

THE SATISFACTORY CONTROL of diabetes with insulin has paradoxically increased the incidence of diabetic retinopathy, for it is apparent from recent analyses that it is the duration of the disease rather than its severity that determines the onset of the retinal changes.

Long-standing mild cases are more likely to show a retinopathy than the severe types of recent onset seen in young people, and the retinal lesions may progress in spite of a well controlled blood-sugar level.

Aneurysm Formation The earliest sign of diabetic retinopathy is an engorgement of the veins. This is followed by degenerative changes in the walls of the terminal vessels, particularly on the venous side, which give way to form minute aneurysms. Fig. 1 shows a flat preparation of the retinal vessels injected with Neoprene. It demonstrates beautifully the saccular dilatations and aneurysms of the capillaries. Usually the aneurysms are formed by the giving way of a small area of the capillary wall with subsequent sacculation. Occasionally a globular aneurysm with afferent and efferent vessels may be found.

These lesions are visible ophthalmoscopically as small red dots scattered about the posterior pole; they are of considerable importance from the diagnostic point of view as they are very rare in any condition other than diabetes. Fig. 2 is a drawing of a relatively early case, showing slight venous engorgement with scattered red dots in the macular region which represent the aneurysms. Previously these red dots had been interpreted as punctate haemorrhages but there is now little doubt that they are really aneurysms.

Haemorrhages and Exudates Sooner or later an aneurysm bursts, giving rise to a small 'blot' haemorrhage. The changes are most marked at the posterior pole and the 'dots' (micro-aneurysms) and 'blots' are accompanied by small yellowish, dry-looking exudates, which may become confluent, as shown in the fundus photograph, Fig. 3. At this stage there may be little visual disturbance unless the macula itself is affected, but later the haemorrhages become more marked and may burst into the vitreous. Such vitreous haemorrhages tend to clear, but recurrence followed by organization of the haemorrhage and retinitis proliferans is only too common. Fig. 4 is a fundus photograph showing a vitreous haemorrhage originating from the region of the disc. The organization of such a haemorrhage causes bands of fibrous tissue in the vitreous which pull on the retina and detach it. Surgery is ineffective in such cases and vision is much reduced or completely lost.

Even if vitreous haemorrhages do not occur, the preponderance of the retinal lesions at the macular area eventually causes a marked diminution of central vision.

Arteriosclerotic changes may be added to the diabetic picture but the predominantly venous and capillary nature of the diabetic process usually makes the diagnosis clear.

51

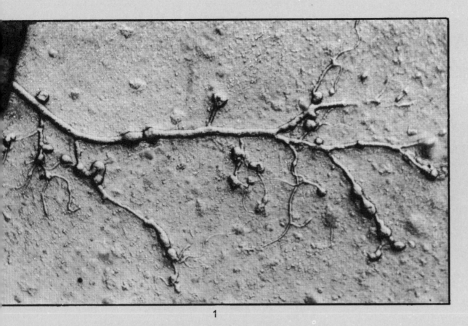

FIG. 1.   NEOPRENE CAST OF RETINAL ANEURYSMS

FIG. 2.   EARLY CHANGES

FIG. 3.   HAEMORRHAGES AND CONFLUENT EXUDATES

FIG. 4.   VITREOUS HAEMORRHAGE

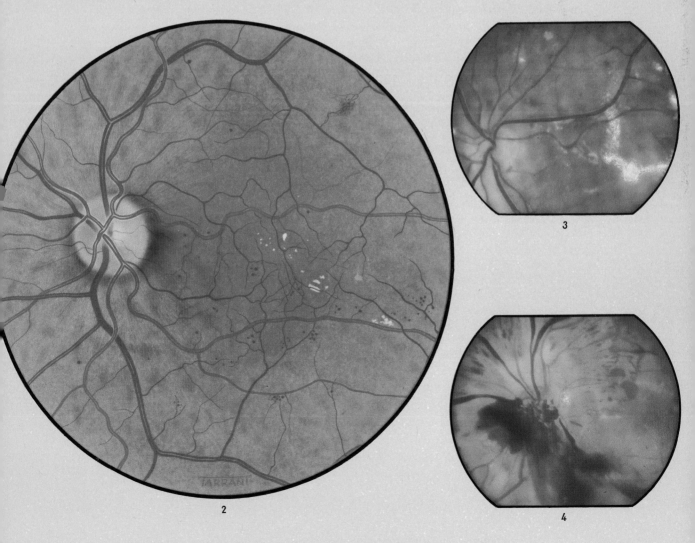

Arterial and Venous Occlusions

Arterial occlusion of the central artery of the retina or one of its branches may be due to spasm, embolus or thrombosis, and unless the obstruction is removed within a few hours, permanent loss of function of that part of the retina supplied by the vessel will result. Sub-acute bacterial endocarditis is the commonest cause of embolic central artery occlusion, while thrombosis may be the result of a true vasculitis or an incident in the course of retinal arteriosclerosis.

However the obstruction is caused, the sequence of events in the retina is the same. The larger arteries are extremely narrowed and the blood column, particularly in the veins, may be broken up into segments, which oscillate with the pulse waves. Meanwhile the retina becomes oedematous and loses its transparency, so that the whole fundus appears much paler than normal except for the macula, which shows up as a bright cherry-red spot standing out prominently against the light background. The disc is also pale. Treatment by the inhalation of amyl nitrite, the retrobulbar injection of acetylcholine and other vasodilators should be instigated immediately.

It is not uncommon to see a vessel supplying the macular region which is not a branch of the central retinal artery but a cilio-retinal artery derived from the short ciliary vessels. In such a case obstruction of the central artery will leave the retina supplied by the cilio-retinal artery unaffected, thus preserving some central vision but with complete loss of the peripheral field.

After a few weeks the retina may regain its normal appearance although the vessels remain small and the disc pale.

Fig. 1 shows the pale central area, with the bright-red spot at the macula and some fragmentation of the blood in the lower nasal vessels. Blockage of the superior temporal branch is shown in Fig. 2. Here the pallor and narrowing of the vessels are confined to the upper temporal area.

Venous thrombosis of the retinal veins is a dreaded complication of vascular disease. It may affect a tributary only, as in Fig. 3, or the central vein itself, as in Figs 4 and 5. The immediate result is a great engorgement of the vessel distal to the block with exaggerated tortuosity as the vessel doubles on itself. The capillaries in the watershed of the vein give way, resulting in a mass of haemorrhages, both superficial and deep. Exudates are also present in the affected area. The optic disc is swollen and the margins become indistinct, but the differentiation from papilloedema due to raised intracranial pressure should be made easily by consideration of the history of sudden visual loss combined with the absence of other signs of raised intracranial pressure.

In time the thrombus canalizes and new vascular channels are formed and the haemorrhages and exudates disappear. The function of the affected retina may improve for some months following the occlusion but central vision is almost always affected if the temporal veins are involved.

An intractable thrombotic glaucoma follows complete central vein thrombosis in some 10 to 20 per cent of cases.

53

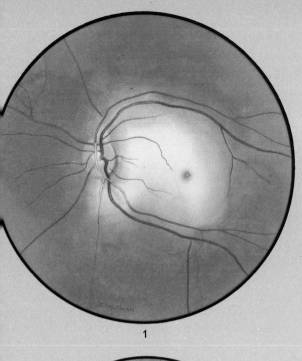

1

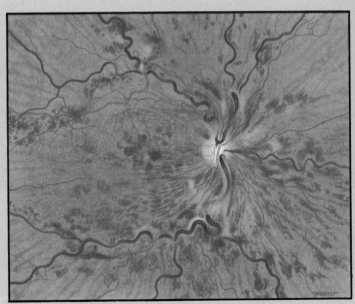

5

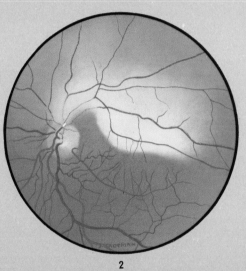

3

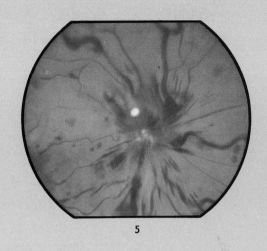

2

FIG. 1.   OCCLUSION OF THE CENTRAL RETINAL ARTERY

FIG. 2.   ARTERIAL BRANCH OCCLUSION

FIG. 3.   VENOUS BRANCH OCCLUSION

FIG. 4.   CENTRAL VEIN THROMBOSIS

FIG. 5.   HAEMORRHAGES AT DISC IN CENTRAL VEIN OCCLUSION

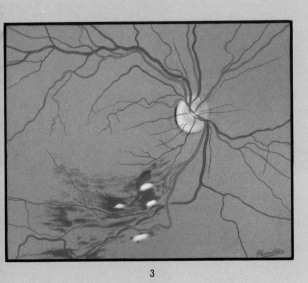

4

Retinal Peri-vasculitis

CHARACTERISTIC RETINAL CHANGES affecting the blood vessels are found in a group of diseases, the pathology of which is still obscure. The most clear-cut clinical entity is Eales's Disease, a chronic retinal periphlebitis occurring in young adults and characterized by recurrent vitreous haemorrhages. Histological examinations have shown the condition to be tuberculous in some cases, but this is not the only cause.

Periphlebitis The condition starts as a patch of inflammation in and around the wall, which shows in the acute stage as a greyish fluffy exudate which may obscure the vein. Scattered lesions of this type may be found all round the periphery of the fundus. Both eyes are affected as a rule but usually one more than the other in the early stages of the disease. Fig. 1 shows the exudates well.

Retinal haemorrhages accompany the acute phase and frequently the blood penetrates into the vitreous completely obscuring the fundus and causing sudden loss of vision. This is usually the symptom which brings the patient for advice. In the early attacks the vitreous may clear completely but later organization of the recurrent haemorrhages may take place, giving rise to retinitis proliferans – an outgrowth of vascular tissue into the vitreous from the disc or retina, illustrated in Fig. 3. This organized tissue may retract and pull on the retina sufficiently to detach it.

The disease tends to regress as the patient gets older and providing there has not been gross vitreous disturbance some vision is retained. Only too often, however, bilateral retinal detachment follows with a hopeless prognosis for vision. Typically, the retinal vein lesions are towards the periphery of the retina (Fig. 2), but there is a group of cases presenting as central vein thrombosis in young adults, which is probably a type of periphlebitis affecting the central vein.

Occasionally an inflammation of the uveal tract complicates the retinal vascular lesions.

Peri-arteritis In contrast to Eales's Disease, in which the veins are predominantly affected, peri-arteritis is relatively rare. Temporal arteritis is a disease of old age in which the temporal arteries of one or both sides become swollen and very tender to touch. It is frequently associated with sudden loss of vision on the affected side or sides. The ophthalmoscopic signs are usually minimal but there may be slight oedema of the disc, though sometimes pallor only is evident. The loss of vision is due to an obliterative arteritis of the nutrient vessels supplying the optic nerve. Occlusion of the central artery of the retina or one of its branches is rare. The prognosis for vision is poor, little improvement occurring in most cases. Fig. 4 is a photograph showing the typical swollen temporal arteries.

In peri-arteritis nodosa, multiple arterial lesions accompanied by haemorrhages and exudates may be seen in the retina. It is a rare condition and the fundus appearance, although suggestive of an arterial disease, is not pathognomonic.

55

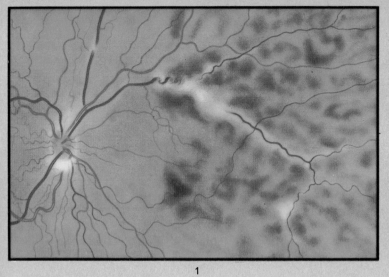

1

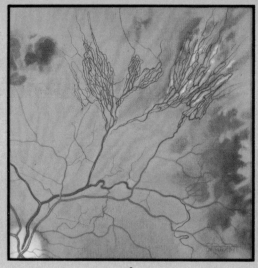

2

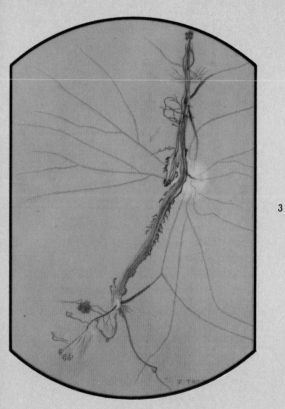

3

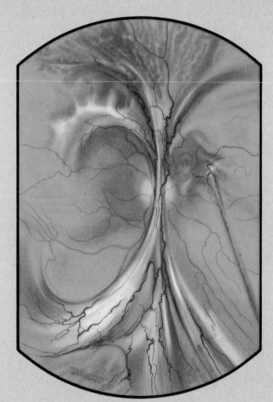

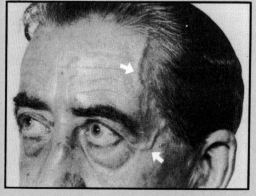

4

FIG. 1.   PERI-VASCULAR EXUDATES

FIG. 2.   PERIPHERAL LESIONS WITH NEW VESSEL FORMATION

FIG. 3.   EARLY AND LATE STAGES OF RETINITIS PROLIFERANS

FIG. 4.   TEMPORAL ARTERITIS

Miscellaneous Systemic Conditions Involving the Retina

Retinopathy of Pregnancy A severe type of hypertensive retinopathy may accompany toxaemia of pregnancy. The onset is sudden, usually during the ninth month. Initially the retinal arteries show transient spasms which are followed by sclerotic changes, scattered haemorrhages and gross exudation. In some cases the retina is detached by the exudate, as shown in the fundus drawing, Fig. 1. In all cases hypertension above 150 mm. Hg systolic and 100 mm. Hg diastolic is present and the retinal changes run parallel with the course of the hypertension. The renal changes are dependent on the hypertension.

Providing the cause of the toxaemia is removed, the prognosis for vision is much more favourable than the ophthalmoscopic picture would suggest, and the retina may reattach itself when the exudate is absorbed.

Renal Retinopathy Whether the retinal changes accompanying severe kidney damage with hypertension are due solely to the vascular changes, or whether some toxic agent is also at work, is not yet decided. The retinal picture is essentially that of vascular sclerosis with haemorrhages and marked retinal oedema, particularly in the macular region, where a 'star' figure is produced. Fig. 2 is a fundus painting showing an incomplete macular star with numerous haemorrhages and soft fluffy exudates.

The distinction between a renal retinopathy and a hypertensive retinopathy is mainly one of degree. In renal retinopathy the marked retinal oedema and masses of 'cotton wool' patches of exudate with very constricted vessels are the diagnostic features.

Anaemia Any severe anaemia may produce retinal changes of the type shown in Fig. 3. The veins are engorged and numerous flame-shaped haemorrhages with pale centres are seen at the posterior pole in relation to the retinal vessels. Some 'woolly' exudates are also present.

Fundus changes are not common after acute traumatic haemorrhages and are more likely to occur following bleeding from medical conditions such as haematemesis, renal haemorrhage and haemoptysis. Recurrent small haemorrhages are more likely to affect vision than a single large loss of blood.

The loss of vision, usually bilateral, may be transient or permanent and the onset may be delayed for some days.

Leucaemia Changes in the fundus are more rare in leucaemia than in anaemia, but pictures similar to those seen in Fig. 4 may occur in any severe type of the former disease. In Fig. 4 (left) the retinal vessels are grossly dilated with occasional haemorrhages. Later the retina looks paler, due to leucocytic infiltration, and the vessel walls become somewhat opaque, almost hiding the blood column, Fig. 4 (right).

Such changes are almost always present in the terminal stage of the disease. Vision is affected if the haemorrhages invade the central area and constriction of the visual fields is another late manifestation.

57

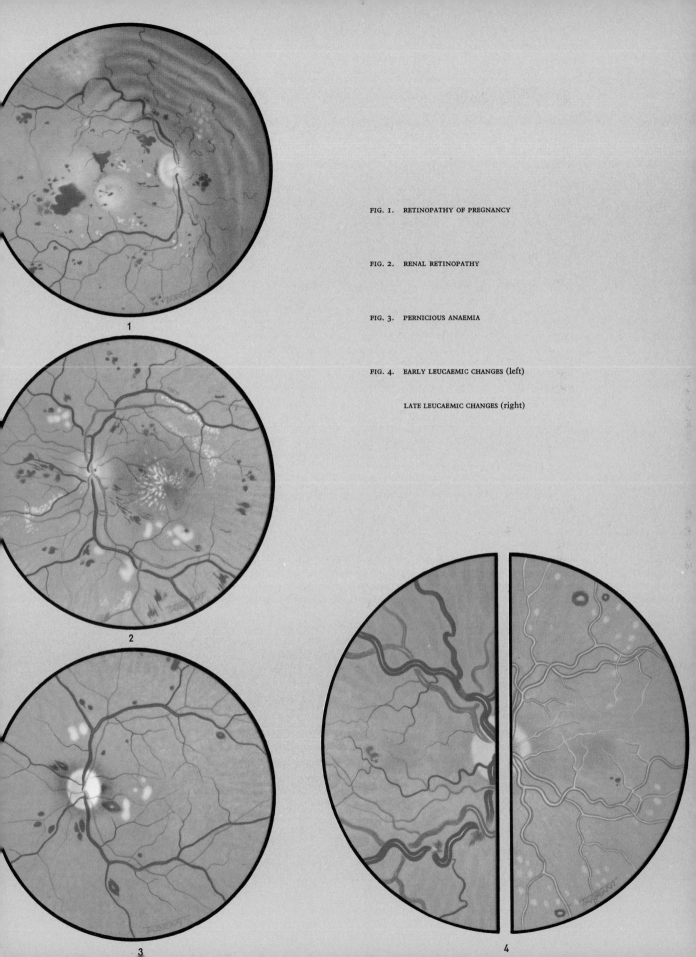

FIG. I.   RETINOPATHY OF PREGNANCY

FIG. 2.   RENAL RETINOPATHY

FIG. 3.   PERNICIOUS ANAEMIA

FIG. 4.   EARLY LEUCAEMIC CHANGES (left)

LATE LEUCAEMIC CHANGES (right)

Optic Disc Changes

Pseudo-papilloedema This congenital variation from the normal appearance of the optic disc is found almost exclusively in small, hypermetropic eyes. It is caused by a heaping up of the nerve fibres combined with an excess of neuroglial tissue, causing the disc to project forward, sometimes to a considerable extent. As seen in Fig. 1, the entire disc is swollen with a greyish and somewhat ill-defined margin. The vessels are of normal calibre and appearance but bend in a curve as they pass from the swollen disc to the retina.

It is important to notice that venous engorgement, haemorrhages and exudates are never present. Frequently the vision cannot be corrected to the normal standard in these cases.

Papilloedema and Optic Neuritis The importance of establishing a diagnosis of papilloedema cannot be overestimated. The fully developed condition is not easily misinterpreted, but minor degrees of swelling may be very difficult to diagnose.

Papilloedema is essentially a passive oedema due to raised intracranial pressure, the first evidence of which is an increased redness of the disc with some blurring of the margins, particularly of its upper and lower parts. The physiological cup becomes filled in and some sheathing of the vessels may be noticed. The veins become congested and the swelling of the disc increases. At this stage the whole margin of the disc becomes indistinct and flame-shaped haemorrhages and exudates begin to appear. In the fully developed condition, shown in Fig. 2, the disc can be seen to be considerably raised above the level of the surrounding retina; the veins are engorged and the vessels dip sharply down to the retina, losing their light reflex as they bend away from the observer.

The oedema spreads to the surrounding retina, particularly towards the macula and may produce a partial macular star.

The appearance of an optic neuritis is very similar to that of papilloedema and the differential diagnosis depends essentially on the absence of raised intracranial pressure and the symptomatology. Papilloedema may have little effect on central vision or the peripheral field, but in optic neuritis the loss of vision is marked and may precede the changes at the disc.

Physiological and Pathological Cupping Most normal optic discs have a central depression and in some eyes this may be sufficiently marked to raise a doubt as to whether the condition is physiological or pathological. In physiological cupping the colour of the disc is normal although the bottom of the cup may be lighter than the edges, and the structure of the lamina cribrosa may be distinguished as a lattice-like pattern. The vessels climb up the edges of the cup but can be seen along their whole course, Fig. 3.

In pathological cupping, on the other hand, the disc is always pale, due to the concomitant optic atrophy. The cup extends the whole width of the disc and a marked parallax can be obtained between the edge of the cup and the bottom where the lamina cribrosa shows clearly, Fig. 4. As the condition is almost always caused by glaucoma, the ocular tension will often be raised in an untreated case.

Optic Atrophy Optic atrophy may follow swelling of the disc or may arise without preceding oedema or inflammation.

The disc is very pale and shows up clearly against the surrounding fundus. The main retinal vessels are narrowed and some degree of cupping is present, due simply to atrophy of the nerve bundles. The lamina cribrosa is often clearly seen.

The atrophy may be limited to one portion of the disc only, as for example, the temporal pallor following an optic neuritis in which the papillomacular bundle of fibres is particularly affected.

59

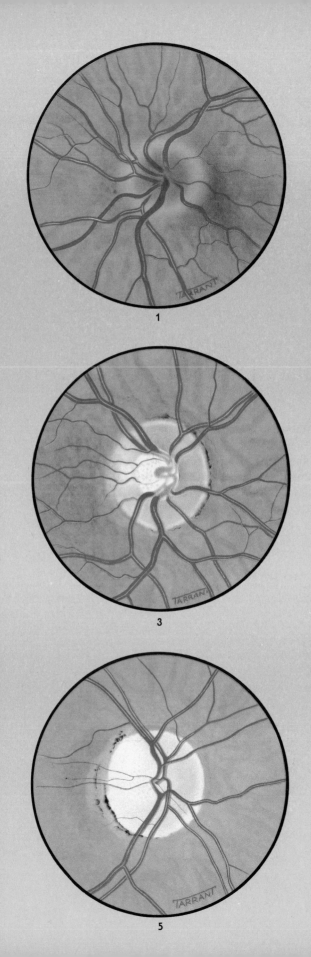

1

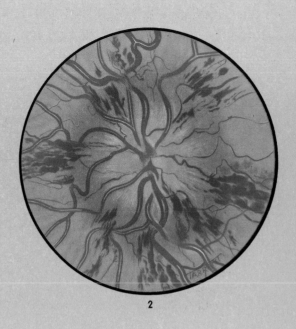

2

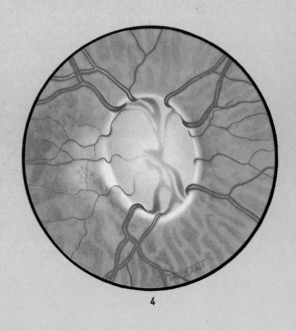

3

FIG. I.   PSEUDO-PAPILLOEDEMA

FIG. 2.   PAPILLOEDEMA

FIG. 3.   PHYSIOLOGICAL CUPPING OF THE DISC

FIG. 4.   EXTREME GLAUCOMATOUS CUPPING OF THE DISC

FIG. 5.   OPTIC ATROPHY

5

4

Congenital Lesions of the Fundus

Albinism There is a very wide variation in the degree of pigmentation of the skin and the uveal tract in normal persons but as far as the eye is concerned, lack of retinal pigment is the criterion of abnormality. It is only when the retinal pigment epithelium is abnormal that symptoms are produced. The condition of albinism is congenital and inherited as a Mendelian recessive.

The eyebrows and lashes are usually white; this combined with narrowing of the palpebral fissures to decrease the amount of light entering the eyes, presents a characteristic clinical appearance. The associated rapid horizontal or rotatory nystagmus may be due to poor central fixation. The iris is a pink-grey colour and in the pupil a red reflex can be seen due to light penetrating the sclera, traversing the depigmented choroid and illuminating the fundus. Fairly high refractive errors are common and vision is always poor, partly due to the scattering of light in the eye and partly due to the poor development and function of the macula in this condition. As shown in Fig. 1 the whole fundus is pale and the individual retinal and choroidal vessels show up clearly against the white sclera. The patients are always photophobic and much can be done to help them by providing dark glasses or tinted contact lenses with an artificial pupil.

Coloboma Colobomata are the result of imperfect closure of the foetal cleft of the optic vesicle in embryonic life and on the extent of this imperfection will depend the extent of the coloboma. It may involve singly or together the iris, ciliary body, choroid, retina and optic nerve.

Fig. 2 is a fundus drawing of a typical coloboma of the retina and choroid. Where the tissues are lacking the sclera shows up as a white area, the gap being bridged by thin, poorly differentiated tissue which may contain some retinal vessels. There is a scotoma in the visual field corresponding to, although usually smaller than, the defective area. Other congenital abnormalities are frequently present.

Opaque Nerve Fibres Medullation of the optic nerve fibres starts centrally, and at birth has normally reached a level immediately behind the lamina cribrosa, where the process stops. Sometimes, however, the process continues after birth (so that the condition is not truly congenital) and the appearance shown in Fig. 3 is produced.

The nerve fibres, which are normally transparent, appear brilliantly white and opaque against the red background of the fundus, and their arcuate course from the disc over the macular region can be clearly traced. The retinal vessels are partly obscured.

Vision is little affected, although there is a partial scotoma corresponding to the area involved.

Conus A white lunate area is commonly seen at the edge of the disc, often with a fringe of pigment along its convex edge. It is due to a gap in the choroid adjacent to the disc and the latter will be found to have the appearance of being tilted about its vertical axis. Astigmatism is usual in these eyes and the vision often cannot be corrected to normal standards.

61

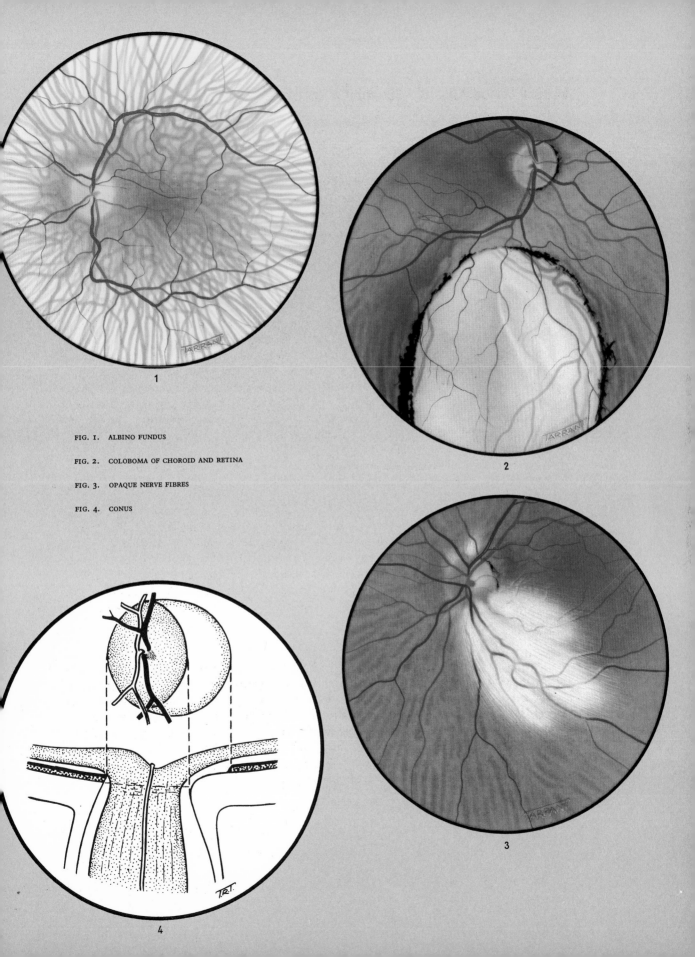

FIG. 1.   ALBINO FUNDUS

FIG. 2.   COLOBOMA OF CHOROID AND RETINA

FIG. 3.   OPAQUE NERVE FIBRES

FIG. 4.   CONUS

Congenital Lesions of the Fundus (contd.)

Choroideremia There is some doubt whether this rare condition is truly congenital or whether it is an abiotrophy of the choroid. It is certainly hereditary, usually as a sex-linked characteristic. It occurs almost always in men and the earliest symptoms are night blindness and field defects. Central vision is not affected until late in the disease. Ophthalmoscopically, as seen in Fig. 1, the choroid is almost entirely absent, except for a patch at the macula and some peripheral areas; here the retinal vessels show up clearly against the white sclera. Scattered pigment deposits may also be seen.

Persistence of the Hyaloid Artery It will be remembered that in embryo the hyaloid artery enters the eye through the upper end of the foetal fissure and extends forward to break up to form the posterior part of the tunica vasculosa lentis which supplies the growing lens with nourishment.

Normally the whole hyaloid system has atrophied before birth, but quite commonly remnants of the hyaloid vessels may be found to persist. A small spot on the posterior capsule of the lens can be seen by the slit-lamp in a large number of adult eyes, marking the termination of the main artery.

In the grosser forms of persistence of the hyaloid artery, a strand of glial tissue containing vessels extends from the centre of the optic disc to the posterior surface of the lens. Such a condition is illustrated in Fig. 2. More usually, a fine thread, which may or may not reach the lens, can be seen extending from the disc.

If the posterior tunica vasculosa lentis persists, a sheet of tissue covers the back of the lens, causing severe obstruction to vision but the milder forms of the abnormality rarely cause symptoms.

Cilio-retinal Vessels The pattern of the normal retinal vessels varies considerably and is of little clinical significance; but occasionally part of the retina is supplied by a vessel derived from the ciliary system. Such a vessel, usually an artery, is called a cilio-retinal vessel. As seen in the drawing, Fig. 3, such vessels appear at the margin of the disc and curve over its edge to supply the adjacent retina. Commonly a vessel of this type goes to the macular region and, should the central retinal artery become blocked, macular vision may be preserved in this event by the unaffected cilio-retinal artery.

Hole in the Optic Disc In this condition an out-pouching of the secondary optic vesicle produces a crater-like hole in the optic disc. The hole is usually oval in shape with the long axis vertical and it may vary in depth from a millimetre or so to a centimetre. It appears bluish-grey in colour, an optical effect probably due to shadows thrown on the floor of the pit. Pathological examination shows that the hole is lined by rudimentary retinal tissue. Retinal vessels sometimes enter the pit and descend to cross the floor before rising and continuing over the disc.

Slight degrees of the deformity produce no symptoms, but field defects and macular lesions have been reported in association with larger craters.

63

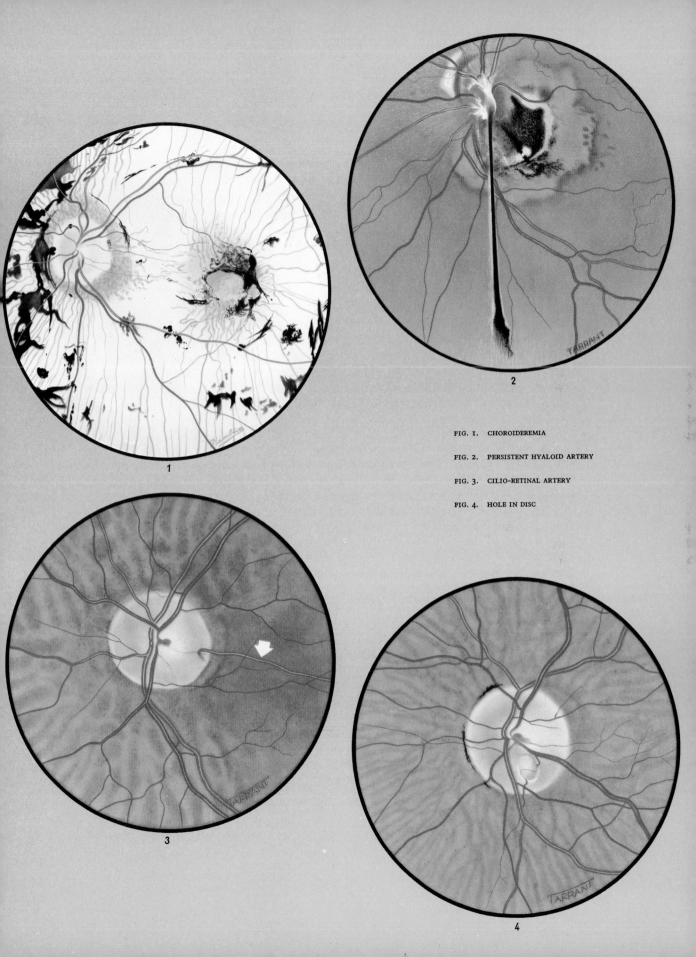

FIG. 1.   CHOROIDEREMIA

FIG. 2.   PERSISTENT HYALOID ARTERY

FIG. 3.   CILIO-RETINAL ARTERY

FIG. 4.   HOLE IN DISC

Haemangiomatosis Retinae

ALTHOUGH THE SYSTEMIC NATURE of haemangiomatosis retinae (or von Hippel-Lindau's disease) may not be recognizable clinically, it is probable that other similar lesions are present in the brain or abdominal viscera in most cases.

The lesions are true angiomata complicated by aneurysm formation and an exudative reaction. A familial incidence can be discovered in about one-fifth of all cases.

Fundus Appearances The clinical appearances are very variable and may range from a single angioma, with its greatly dilated afferent and efferent vessels, to a gross exudative retinal detachment with many enormously dilated vessels, haemorrhages and exudates involving the whole fundus. The commonest appearance, shown in Fig. 1, is of enormously dilated vessels extending from the optic disc and ending in an angiomatous cystic tumour. Fig. 2 is a fundus photograph showing the dilated vessels. Haemorrhages and exudates occur around the lesion and frequently the retina becomes detached by the gross exudation. The detachment eventually becomes complete with tortuous, greatly enlarged vessels coursing over the surface. Secondary glaucoma and degeneration of the eye may follow.

Fig. 3 shows another form of haemangiomatosis consisting of miliary aneurysms of the retinal vessels combined with retinal degeneration. Occasionally the changes are limited to the macular region but more usually the whole retina is involved. The exudation increases and serious retinal damage is caused. In Fig. 3 can be seen several globular aneurysms of branches of the inferior temporal artery with exudates near the macula. Similar lesions but without exudates are seen peripherally and the veins show localized fusiform swellings.

Single Angiomata Single angiomata not associated with systemic lesions sometimes occur at the optic disc. They show as well-defined reddish tumours projecting forward from the disc. The margins may be fairly smooth, as in the case illustrated in Fig. 4, or the tumour may have a 'raspberry' appearance, with a nodular surface.

The vision is not affected in the earlier stages but traction on the retina may diminish central vision later. Extension of the tumour takes place slowly and the final prognosis is not good.

Treatment Haemangiomatosis is difficult to treat but the application of diathermy or radiation therapy to localized areas of tumour formation has met with some success. If the tumour is not destroyed, haemorrhages eventually take place and glaucoma ensues, with final destruction of the eye.

65

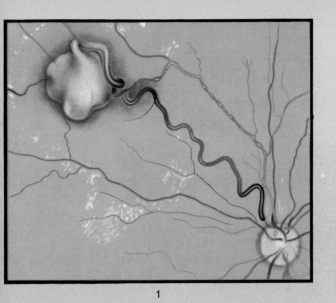

1

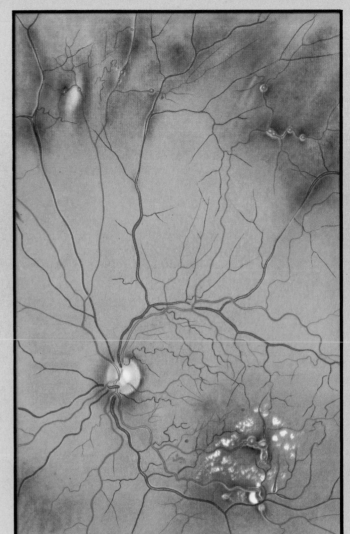

2

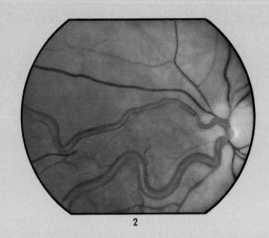

3

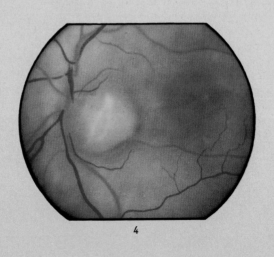

4

FIG. 1.   SINGLE HAEMANGIOMA

FIG. 2.   GROSS DILATATION OF VESSELS

FIG. 3.   MILIARY ANEURYSM FORMATION

FIG. 4.   HAEMANGIOMA AT DISC

Trauma to the Posterior Segment

TRAUMA TO THE EYE may be roughly divided into concussion injuries and perforating injuries; whereas the fundus appearances naturally vary considerably, some typical changes may occur in each group.

Concussion Injuries These injuries follow blows on the eye from large objects such as a fist or tennis ball. The shock-wave travels through the fluid media of the eye and produces its main effects at the posterior pole. The retina, and in particular the macular region, like all highly developed tissue, is more susceptible to damage than the choroid. Comparatively trivial blows with little external evidence of injury may cause permanent macular lesions with diminished central vision – a good reason for giving a guarded prognosis in all ocular injuries.

Commotio Retinae is the term used for oedema of the macular region following a concussion injury. The retina at the posterior pole becomes slightly opaque and has a milky sheen, the macula showing as a bright red spot, Fig. 1. The oedema subsides but is often followed by pigmentary or cystic macular changes. The latter give the appearance of a sharply defined 'hole' at the macula, Fig. 2; but microscopic examination has shown that the condition is really cystic. Central vision is markedly affected.

In more severe cases of concussion injury the choroid may be torn, as shown in Figs 3 and 4, the tears appearing as yellowish streaks with some pigment disturbance at the edges, roughly concentric with the optic disc.

Retinal tears may also occur in such injuries and they are very likely to be followed by detachment. This complication will be described in a later section. Frequently, vitreous haemorrhages obscure the fundus picture in the more severe injuries and the extent of the retinal and choroidal damage can only be assessed when the haemorrhage has been absorbed.

Perforating Injuries The grosser penetrating wounds caused by large objects usually cause such disorganization of the eye that the fundus cannot be seen, but frequently a small metallic foreign body may penetrate the globe, apparently causing remarkably little disturbance. The patient may feel little or no pain and unless the anterior chamber is lost, the lens injured or haemorrhage takes place in the eye, the sight may not be immediately affected. It is not uncommon for the presence of the foreign body to be unsuspected for days, weeks or even years, until visual changes bring the patient for examination.

The amount of damage caused by the entry of the foreign body depends on its size and route. In hammer-and-chisel injuries, in which a small flake from the hammer-head flies back into the eye, the fragment usually penetrates the cornea, crosses the anterior chamber and goes through the iris or pupil and the lens. It may, however, enter at the limbus and pass through the zonule of the lens into the vitreous chamber. Its subsequent course depends on its propulsive force, but frequently it comes to rest embedded in the retina near the posterior pole.

The fundus drawing, Fig. 5, shows such a foreign body embedded in the retina with consequent pigmentary changes; the vitreous disturbance caused by its passage is clearly seen.

67

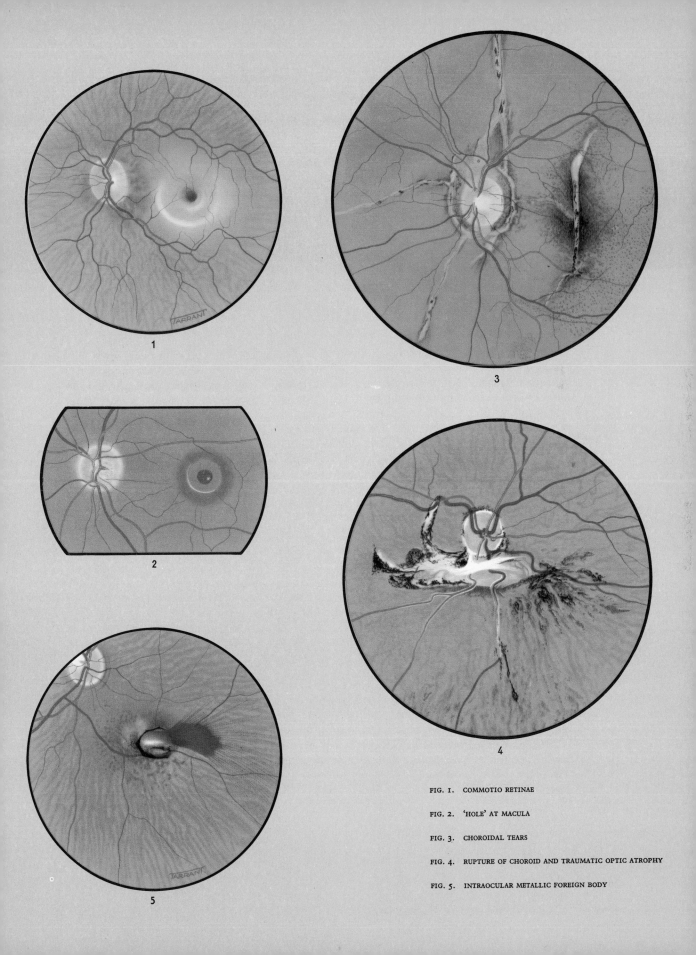

FIG. 1. COMMOTIO RETINAE

FIG. 2. 'HOLE' AT MACULA

FIG. 3. CHOROIDAL TEARS

FIG. 4. RUPTURE OF CHOROID AND TRAUMATIC OPTIC ATROPHY

FIG. 5. INTRAOCULAR METALLIC FOREIGN BODY

Choroiditis

AS THE OUTER LAYERS of the retina are dependent on the choroid for their blood supply, any inflammation of the choroid is bound to affect the retina, either directly or indirectly, although this may not be obvious ophthalmoscopically.

Aetiology As in the case of inflammatory lesions of the rest of the uveal tract, the aetiology of the condition is often in doubt. Certain diseases are known to produce characteristic choroidal lesions, for example, tuberculosis, syphilis and toxoplasmosis, but a large number of cases in which the cause is doubtful remain, which is variously attributed to focal infection, virus infections or bacterial hypersensitivity.

Tuberculous Choroiditis Tuberculous lesions of the choroid are usually caused by the actual invasion of the tissue with *Mycobacterium tuberculosis*. The resulting lesion will depend on the number of infecting organisms and their virulence, and the resistance or specific immunity of the host. The fundus picture may thus vary from the miliary tubercles, seen in the terminal stages of miliary tuberculosis and tuberculous meningitis, to a solitary patch of chronic choroiditis occurring in an otherwise apparently healthy individual. Rarely, a tumour-like tuberculoma may occur.

Fig. 1 is a fundus drawing of a typical miliary type of tuberculous choroiditis. Round, yellowish spots are scattered over the posterior pole, particularly in the neighbourhood of the disc. Their appearance in a case of tuberculous meningitis is evidence of a severe infection.

The fundus photograph, Fig. 2, shows a large patch of healed choroiditis due to tuberculosis. The affected area of choroid has atrophied, and pigment has conglomerated into an irregular dark mass. This is the typical end-appearance of any focal choroiditis and could not be ascribed to tuberculosis on the fundus change alone.

Syphilitic Choroiditis In the acquired disease, syphilitic choroiditis may be indistinguishable from chronic disseminated choroiditis due to other causes, but in the congenital disease a typical appearance may be presented. It is usually described as a 'pepper-and-salt' fundus, wherein the entire fundus is dusted with innumerable bluish pigmented spots, between which lie rounded depigmented areas of yellowish-red colour. The condition remains unchanged throughout life, Fig. 3.

Fig. 4 shows the typical appearance of an old disseminated choroiditis which might be syphilitic or be caused by any of the aetiological factors previously mentioned.

Non-specific Choroiditis Fig. 5 is a fundus drawing of a solitary patch of choroiditis in the acute stage. There is usually some vitreous haze, due to the presence of an inflammatory reaction, causing the symptom of mistiness of vision which brings the patient for advice.

The lesion appears as a white fluffy patch with indefinite margins and over which retinal vessels may course. When healing takes place the choroid undergoes atrophy, leaving a pale clear-cut area with pigment heaped up round the edges.

69

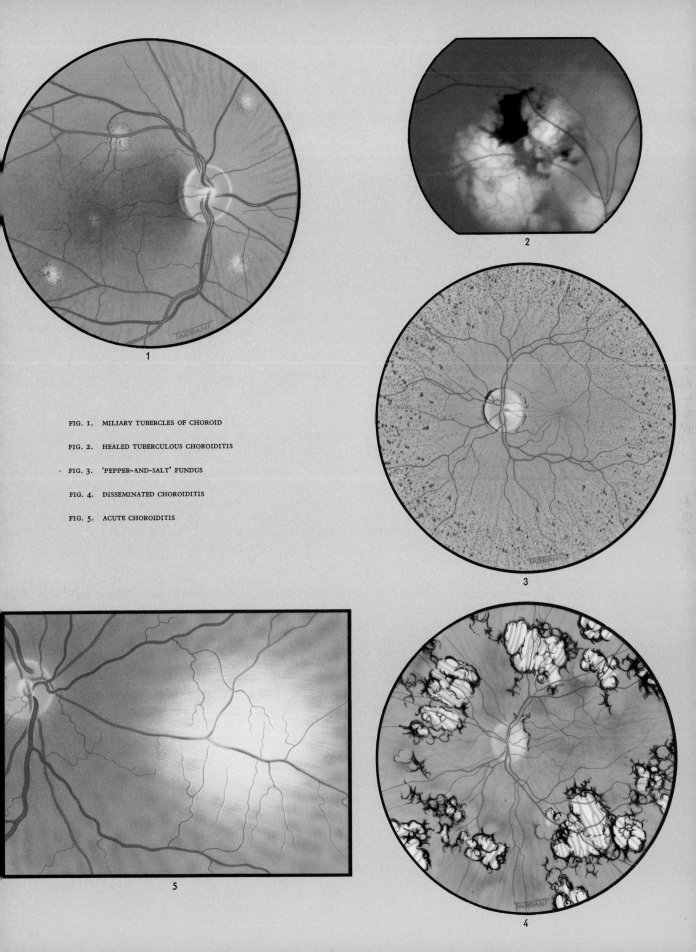

FIG. 1.   MILIARY TUBERCLES OF CHOROID

FIG. 2.   HEALED TUBERCULOUS CHOROIDITIS

FIG. 3.   'PEPPER-AND-SALT' FUNDUS

FIG. 4.   DISSEMINATED CHOROIDITIS

FIG. 5.   ACUTE CHOROIDITIS

Toxoplasmosis

ALTHOUGH THE TOXOPLASMA ORGANISM was first discovered in 1908 by Nicolle and Manceau, reports of human infection remained rare for forty years. It is primarily a disease of rodents, although sporadic infections have been recorded in domestic animals including the dog and the fowl. How the organism is transmitted to man is not yet known.

The Organism   The organism is a protozoon and probably reproduces inside the cells of the host tissue. In its 'free' and pathogenic form it is a slender lunate or slightly curved body becoming increasingly globular with age. It is also found in multi-nuclear clumps or 'cysts' probably representing aggregations of immature organisms.

Toxoplasma are demonstrated most readily in sections of heart, lung, muscle and testis as well as in the brain and eye, but they may also be recovered in living patients from the cerebrospinal fluid.

The commonest human infection occurs in infants, causing a severe encephalomyelitis, either before birth or in early post-natal life. It is characterized by convulsions, spastic deformities, splenomegaly and hepatomegaly and bilateral choroido-retinitis. The eye changes are usually present in the congenital or neo-natal disease and are characterized by a bilateral choroiditis affecting particularly the macular region, but often accompanied by peripheral lesions. Microphthalmos and other congenital defects may be present and nystagmus is usual when the macula is affected. It is probable that many of the cases previously labelled 'coloboma of the macula' were in fact healed choroidal lesions of this aetiology.

Fundus Appearances   The fundus lesions may show a striking similarity in the two eyes. A pale atrophic area surrounded by pigmentary changes is seen at both maculae, sometimes with similar lesions at the periphery. Any focal choroiditis may produce a similar appearance but the site and symmetry of the lesions and their congenital or neo-natal incidence are pathognomonic of toxoplasmosis. Histological examination of the eyes shows areas of acute round-celled infiltration of the choroid and retina with a marked tendency to necrosis. The focal nature of the lesion is shown by the sharp margin between normal and inflamed tissues. The parasite has been demonstrated in the inflamed areas. Brain sections show similar granulomatous changes, and here the necrosis is followed by calcification.

Fig. 1 is a fundus photograph showing a typical lesion at the macula, and Fig. 2 shows a more peripheral lesion in the other eye. Some degree of optic atrophy may be present, and this can be seen in Fig. 4 – a fundus painting of a patient whose other eye is illustrated in Fig. 3. Other typical appearances are shown in Figs 5 and 6.

The brain lesions end in multiple areas of calcification which can be shown by x-rays and are an aid to diagnosis. Several laboratory tests are available, including a cytoplasm-modifying dye test and a complement-fixation test.

Fresh infection of adults has now been reported, and although most of the acquired cases have not shown ocular lesions, a few cases of choroiditis have given serological reactions typical of toxoplasmosis.

71

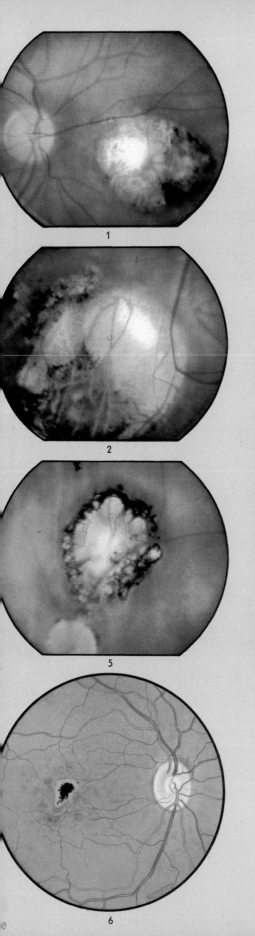

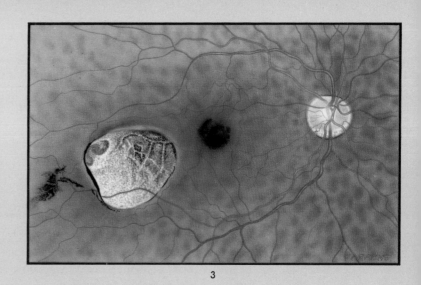

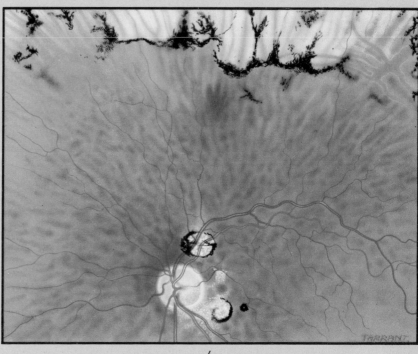

FIG. 1. TYPICAL MACULAR LESION

FIG. 2. PERIPHERAL LESION

FIG. 3.
FIG. 4. } BILATERAL LESIONS WITH OPTIC ATROPHY LEFT EYE

FIG. 5. FOCAL TOXOPLASMIC CHOROIDITIS

FIG. 6. PIGMENTED SCAR OF HEALED LESION

Neoplasms of the Posterior Segment

PIGMENTED TUMOURS of the choroid constitute the largest group of intra-ocular neoplasms; they may be benign or malignant.

Benign Melanoma of the Choroid (Naevus) Choroidal naevi occur relatively frequently but are only discovered on ophthalmoscopical examination and do not give rise to symptoms. They appear at the posterior pole of the eye as flat blue or greyish patches, usually about the same size as the disc. The retinal vessels course normally across them and the overlying retina is not raised or detached. This appearance is well illustrated in Fig. 1.

No treatment is required but the patient should be re-examined at intervals, as occasionally a naevus may eventually become the site of a malignant melanoma.

Malignant Melanoma of the Choroid is a disease of middle life. The symptoms are commonly those of a retinal detachment and the usual history is that a 'shadow' obscures part of the visual field. If, however, the tumour originates at or near to the macula, a disturbance of central vision will take place early.

The tumour starts as a flat infiltration of the choroid, but when it bursts through Bruch's membrane, which separates the choroid from the retina, it grows more freely, pushing the retina before it. Fig. 3 is a section of an eye containing such a tumour and shows the constriction at the 'neck' of the tumour where it has penetrated Bruch's membrane. If left untreated the retina becomes completely detached, glaucoma supervenes and extra-ocular extension and metastases occur.

In early cases, before the detachment becomes extensive, the tumour may be seen ophthalmoscopically as shown in Fig. 2; but not infrequently the detachment is sufficiently extensive to hide the tumour from view (Fig. 5). The differential diagnosis in such cases can be very difficult. There will be no retinal tear and the usual predisposing features of a simple detachment – myopia or injury – are unlikely to be present. Transillumination of the eye is often helpful and recently radio-active phosphorus has been used to assist in the diagnosis.

The degree of pigmentation of the tumour varies greatly from the so-called leucosarcoma with minimum pigmentation (Fig. 4) to a darkly pigmented growth but this feature is of little importance in assessing the degree of malignancy.

Direct extension of the tumour through the channels in the sclera, formed by the perforating vessels and nerves, occurs relatively early. Extra-ocular metastases may also occur early and may even lead the patient to seek advice before the primary lesion has been noticed.

The metastases are blood-borne and do not affect the lymph nodes. The liver is by far the commonest organ affected and as the metastases may not be clinically evident for many years, prognosis is always uncertain. The microscopical appearance of the tumour tissue gives some guide to its malignancy; tumours composed of spindle-cells with a high reticulin content have a better prognosis than tumours containing cells of a more anaplastic type with a low reticulin content.

The treatment of malignant melanoma of the choroid is enucleation of the eye as soon as possible after the diagnosis has been made. If there is any evidence of extra-ocular extension, exenteration of the orbit must be considered, but as it is relatively rare for orbital recurrences to take place, irradiation of the orbit is a sufficient safeguard in most cases. The survival rate after enucleation is difficult to assess but is probably in the neighbourhood of 50 per cent for a five-year period.

73

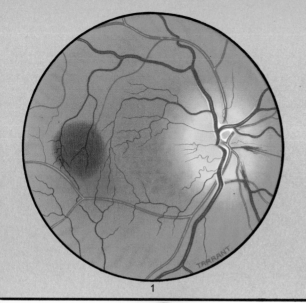

1

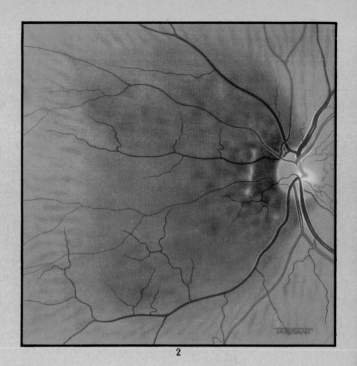

2

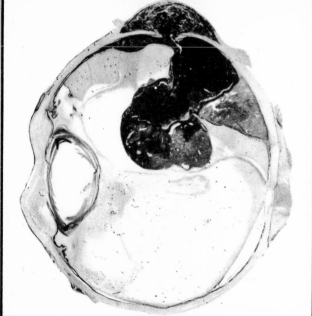

3

FIG. 1.   CHOROIDAL NAEVUS

FIG. 2.   EARLY MALIGNANT MELANOMA OF THE CHOROID

FIG. 3.   SECTION OF AN EYE SHOWING ADVANCED
          MALIGNANT MELANOMA

FIG. 4.   NON-PIGMENTED LEUCOSARCOMA

FIG. 5.   TUMOUR CAUSING WIDESPREAD DETACHMENT
          OF THE RETINA

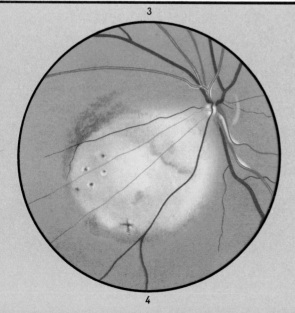

4

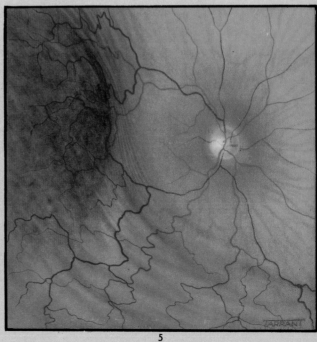

5

Neoplasms of the Posterior Segment (cont.)

Retinoblastoma The pathology of this tumour is of considerable interest. Formerly called a 'glioma' of the retina, it is now recognized as a congenital tumour arising from cell rests of the primitive neuro-ectoderm which forms the optic vesicle. One or both eyes are affected and multiple origins of growth are usual. It develops most commonly in the first two years of life but a later onset is not unknown.

Retinoblastoma shows a definite hereditary tendency but the mode of transmission is irregular and sporadic cases are in the majority. The risk of a second child of normal parents being affected is about 1 per cent but the children of an affected parent who has survived the disease show a much higher incidence rate.

The tumour arises from the inner or outer nuclear layers of the retina and either grows into the vitreous or into the subretinal space, causing extensive retinal detachment. In either case the whole vitreous chamber eventually fills with new growth, as seen in Fig. 3.

As the disease occurs in infants, the first evidence is usually a yellow reflex in the pupil – the so-called 'amaurotic cat's eye' (Fig. 2). The early stages of the tumour are rarely seen except in the second, less affected eye, of bilateral cases. Fig. 1 shows such a lesion in a child whose other eye had been removed. In this case the tumour appears to arise from a single area and the creamy mass protruding into the vitreous is characteristic.

In the late stages, metastatic nodules appear on the iris and in the anterior chamber.

The differential diagnosis includes congenital abnormalities such as persistence of the primary vitreous, inflammatory conditions and possibly retrolental fibroplasia, although in the latter condition the history of prematurity and oxygen therapy will be obtained.

The growth spreads initially by direct extension through the sclera and along the optic nerve, cerebral involvement being the commonest cause of death. Metastatic spread via the bloodstream does occur but is more common after extra-ocular extension has involved the orbital contents.

Treatment is enucleation with as long a piece of optic nerve as possible and exenteration of the orbit if extra-ocular extension is discovered. In bilateral cases, when the second eye contains only a small tumour, radiotherapy to this eye is justified, as retinoblastoma is usually very radio-sensitive, providing a sufficient dose can be applied to the whole tumour.

Secondary Tumours The eye is not a common site for metastatic deposits from tumours in other organs of the body, although no doubt small lesions occur in the terminal stages of carcinomatosis but are unnoticed.

If they do occur it is usually in the choroid at the posterior pole and the breast is the commonest site of the primary lesion. Occasionally the uveal tumour may be the first evidence of the primary lesion, the visual disturbance bringing the patient for advice before the systemic symptoms. Clinically the tumour appears as a circumscribed raised yellowish area at the posterior pole associated with some degree of retinal detachment, as seen in Fig. 4. It may spread forwards as far as the ciliary body, as shown in the section in Fig. 5, but rarely penetrates into the vitreous.

Such tumours are part of a generalized carcinomatosis with an inevitable fatal outcome. Radiotherapy and bilateral removal of the suprarenals may secure temporary recession.

75

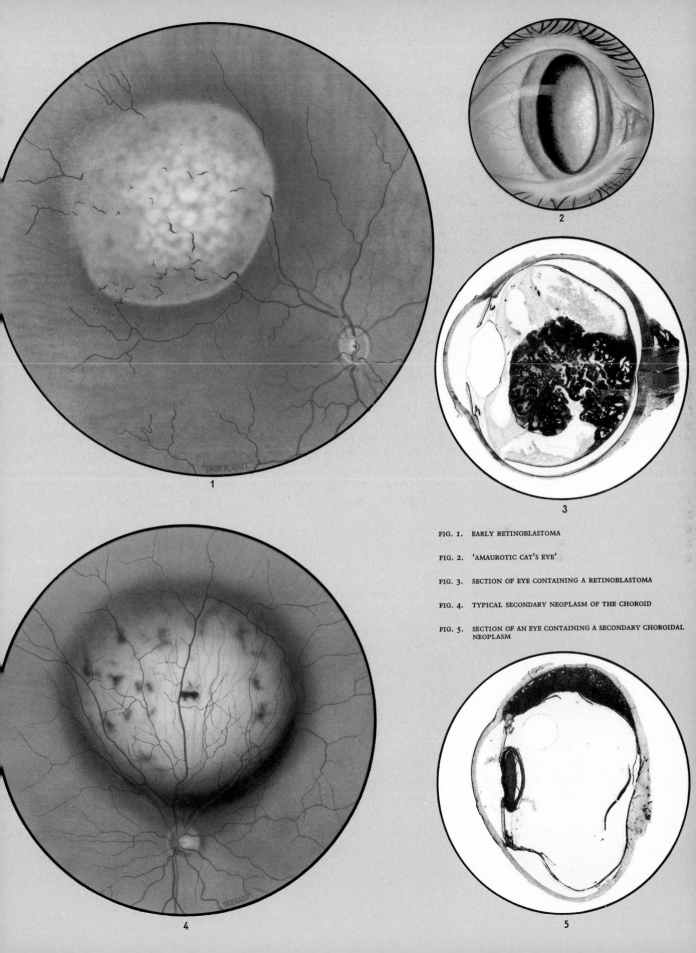

FIG. 1.   EARLY RETINOBLASTOMA

FIG. 2.   'AMAUROTIC CAT'S EYE'

FIG. 3.   SECTION OF EYE CONTAINING A RETINOBLASTOMA

FIG. 4.   TYPICAL SECONDARY NEOPLASM OF THE CHOROID

FIG. 5.   SECTION OF AN EYE CONTAINING A SECONDARY CHOROIDAL
NEOPLASM

Retinal Detachment

THE PIGMENT EPITHELIUM of the retina is firmly adherent to the choroid but only loosely attached to the layer of rods and cones except at the disc and peripherally at the ora serrata. The condition known as retinal detachment is in reality a separation of the main retina from the pigment epithelium, thus reforming the space originally present in the primary optic vesicle.

The causes of this retinal separation are many and the mechanism involved is often obscure. Detachments secondary to neoplasms or exudative lesions of the choroid, as described in previous sections, are easier to understand than the so-called idiopathic type to be discussed here. It is probable that the fundamental change is a small area of mild inflammation or degeneration of the thinner peripheral retina to which vitreous becomes adherent. Movement of the eye or trauma causes the vitreous to pull on the retina, thus creating a tear or hole. When this has happened fluid vitreous can pass through the hole and strip the retina off the pigment layer. In some cases it is possible to see a small area of retina suspended in the vitreous over the site of the hole; in others a V-shaped tag of retina is pulled up, giving rise to an 'arrowhead' type of tear as depicted in Fig. 1. The upper temporal region is the most common site.

Myopia is a common predisposing factor and it has been estimated that two-thirds of all idiopathic detachments occur in myopic eyes. As myopia is usually a bilateral condition it follows that if a detachment has occurred in one eye the other eye is also liable to be affected. The association of detachment with myopia is probably due to the stretching and thinning of the coats of the eye associated with the peripheral degenerative areas and the fluid vitreous so commonly found in short-sighted eyes. Trauma, which may be quite trivial, is a frequent precipitating factor.

The history is often quite typical. The patient notices flashes of light in part of the visual field – usually in the nasal area – due to the adherent vitreous pulling on the retina during movements of the eye. Days or weeks later, when the retina starts to detach, a shadow appears in the field corresponding to the affected region. The lower retina is most likely to be detached as the subretinal fluid sinks by the influence of gravity. Sometimes the patient is not aware of anything wrong until the macular region becomes detached, causing loss of central vision. Ophthalmoscopic examination will reveal an area of the retina which is thrown into folds and has a greyish reflex instead of the clear red of the normal retina. The blood-vessels should be carefully examined – they can be seen to follow the retinal folds in the detached area and appear darker than normal and devoid of their central reflex. Slight movements of the eye may elicit corresponding movements of the detached retina.

Some vitreous disturbance is always present and may be sufficiently marked to make examination of the fundus difficult.

It is probable that a hole is present in all cases but it may be very difficult to locate, either because it is at the extreme periphery or because it is hidden in a fold of retina. Sometimes a large arc of retina tears away from the ora serrata, producing a dialysis as illustrated in Fig. 2 which contrasts with the 'arrowhead' type of tear having small areas of thinned retina surrounding it, as shown in Fig. 1. The folding and greyish reflex with the dark blood-vessels are well shown in this fundus painting.

77

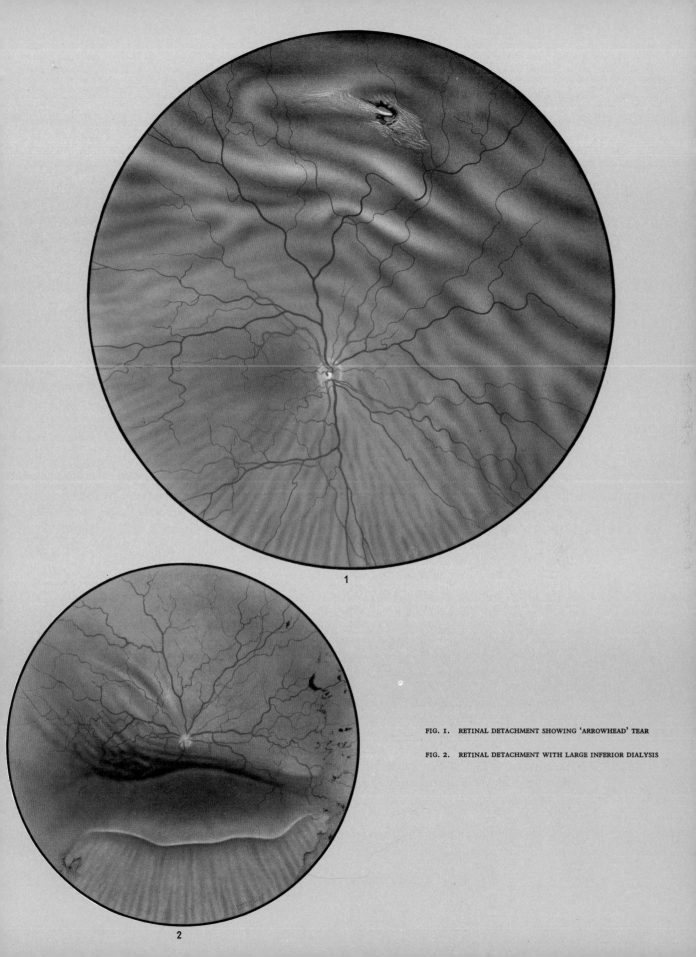

FIG. 1. RETINAL DETACHMENT SHOWING 'ARROWHEAD' TEAR

FIG. 2. RETINAL DETACHMENT WITH LARGE INFERIOR DIALYSIS

Exudative Retinitis or Coats's Disease

THE ESSENTIAL CHARACTERISTIC of this somewhat ill-defined group of lesions is massive exudation in or beneath the retina.

Clinical Aspect This condition is seen in children and young adults, particularly in males. It is normally uniocular, is insidious in onset and slow in progress. In the early stages flecks of deep retinal exudate appear scattered widely over the fundus and, as the disease progresses, these conglomerate to form a subretinal mass. Coats originally described changes in the blood-vessels, especially in the veins, as characteristic of the later stages, but these are not always seen. Such vascular changes consist of loops, twists and dilatations of the vessels, together with many small aneurysms associated with sparse superficial haemorrhages; a considerable spattering of cholesterol crystals is often found in the retina.

In some cases the condition appears to be self-limiting, although an organized area remains in the fundus indefinitely. In the majority of cases, however, the subretinal exudate leads to the development of a retinal detachment with much gliosis; the intra-ocular picture may thus be described as a 'pseudo-glioma' and the condition may end in a complicated glaucoma necessitating enucleation of the eye.

There is no familial tendency; nor do vascular or other lesions occur elsewhere in the body. It has been described as a stage of retinal haemangioblastoma (von Hippel-Lindau's disease) but the isolated involvement of the eye as well as the absence of any neoplastic vascular changes in the retina distinguish the two conditions. The aetiology is unknown and is probably varied. Coats considered the condition to be primarily of haemorrhagic origin; even if the exudation is not based on deep retinal haemorrhages, the common and striking vascular changes would seem to be a more likely aetiological factor than other suggestions such as a toxic-inflammatory state.

No adequate treatment is known; neither diathermy-coagulation nor radiotherapy – both of which may be of value in haemangiomatosis – is effective.

Fig. 1 shows an early stage of the disease with flecking of deep exudate and vascular abnormalities including the characteristic groups and chains of small aneurysms.

Figs 2, 3 and 4 show the varying stages in the development of subretinal masses, from any one of which may suddenly appear a retinal detachment with progressive intra-ocular disorganization.

Pathology The essential pathological finding is a gross disturbance of the retinal structures affecting particularly the deeper layers where albuminous fluid collects to form the subretinal exudate. In both the retina and the exudate, masses of bladder-cells typical of the condition are seen. Changes in the retinal vessels with perivasculitis may be present in some cases while in others both haemorrhage and vascular lesions are absent. In all early cases the pigment layer and the choroid appear normal, but in the later stages some proliferation of the pigment is common.

79

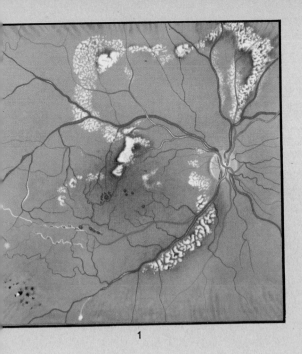

1

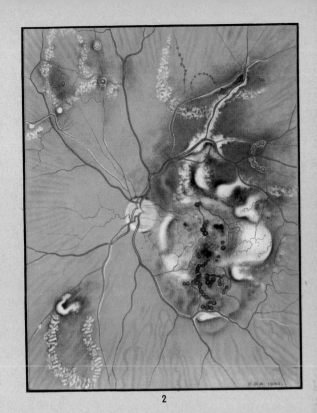

2

FIG. 1.   EARLY STAGE

FIG. 2.   MARKED ANEURYSM FORMATION

FIG. 3.   WIDESPREAD EXUDATION

FIG. 4.   CONGLOMERATE SUBRETINAL MASS

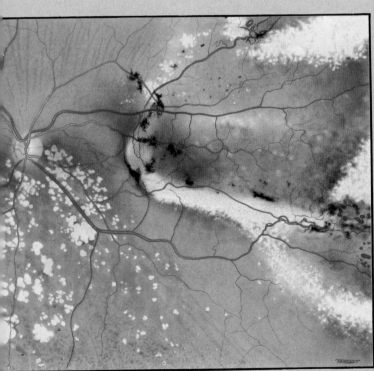

3

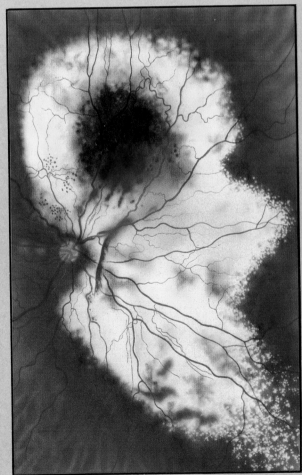

4

Retinitis Pigmentosa

THIS INTERESTING RETINAL CONDITION is a primary degeneration of the neuro-epithelium, accompanied by a widespread pigment disturbance, narrowing of the vessels and optic atrophy. The aetiology is unknown. The condition is hereditary, although the type of transmission varies and sporadic cases occur in which no family history can be obtained. It is important to attempt to determine the type of transmission in each case so that advice can be given on the likelihood of offspring being affected.

If the disease occurs as a dominant characteristic, half the children of an affected person are likely to exhibit the condition. Consanguinity is an important factor in the incidence of the recessive type. Sex-linkage is common, males exhibiting the fully developed condition, whereas the female carriers who are symptomless may nevertheless show a curious increase in reflection from the fundus, somewhat reminiscent of the tapetal reflex of the cat.

Other defects of a degenerative nature may be encountered; thus the association of pigmentary degeneration of the retina with obesity, polydactyly, hypogenitalism and mental retardation constitutes the Laurence-Moon-Biedl syndrome.

The earliest symptom is relative night blindness, which may be first noticed in childhood and is due to the depression of function of the rods which subserve scotopic vision. The degeneration is bilateral, first affecting the equatorial region and producing a ring scotoma in the visual fields. The scotoma gradually spreads out towards the periphery and in towards fixation, until only a small central field remains. Although the acuity of central vision may be quite good the patient is very severely handicapped by the gross field loss. Finally, in middle age the remaining field is lost and not uncommonly cataract develops. Fig. 5 is a composite chart of the visual fields showing a typical ring scotoma on the left, which in the right-hand chart has progressed to leave only a small central area, sometimes described as a 'tubular' field.

The fundus picture is striking in an advanced case. The optic disc is pale and waxy in appearance, the retinal vessels are markedly narrowed and may appear as mere threads. The typical spidery pigment deposits, which have been likened to the Haversian systems in bone, are scattered widely over the peripheral retina. The pigment is frequently found lying along the wall of the veins, as is clearly shown in the fundus photograph (Fig. 2). This migration of pigment from the retinal pigmentary epithelium allows the choroid to be seen more clearly, so that a tessellated pattern and individual choroidal vessels can be seen (Fig. 3).

In an early case the pigment is only present in the equatorial region, while the extreme periphery and central areas appear normal (Fig. 4).

Treatment is very disappointing. The disease is subject to remissions which may coincide with some particular therapy, giving rise to false hopes of improvement, but prophylaxis on eugenic lines gives the best hope of eradicating the condition.

81

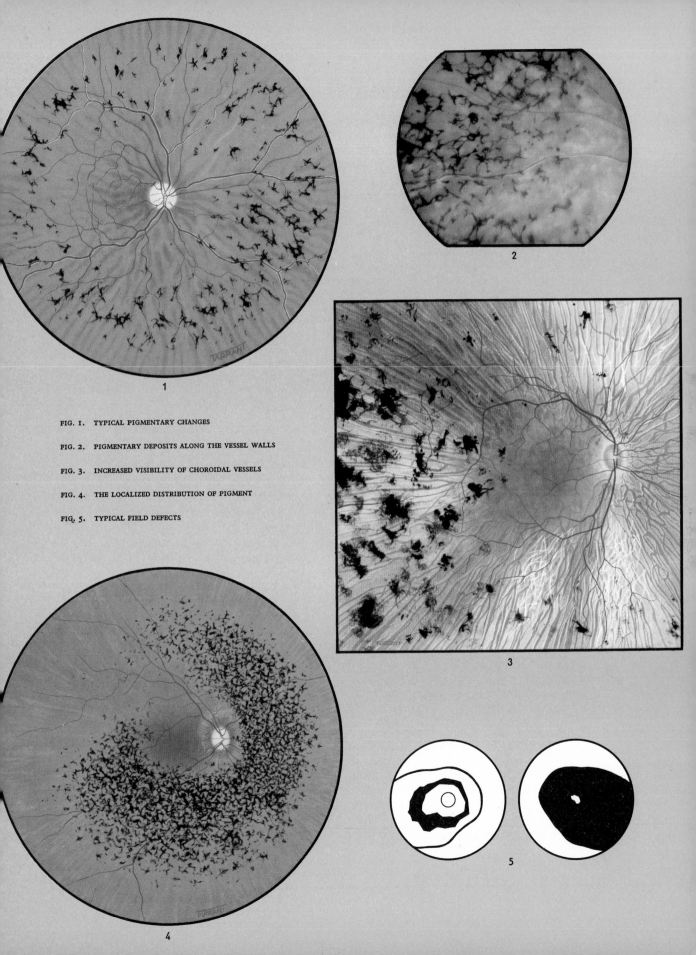

FIG. I. TYPICAL PIGMENTARY CHANGES

FIG. 2. PIGMENTARY DEPOSITS ALONG THE VESSEL WALLS

FIG. 3. INCREASED VISIBILITY OF CHOROIDAL VESSELS

FIG. 4. THE LOCALIZED DISTRIBUTION OF PIGMENT

FIG. 5. TYPICAL FIELD DEFECTS

Heredo-Macular Degenerations

TWO GROUPS of familial macular lesions are represented by these fundus pictures. The first group is not associated with lesions in other systems of the body but in the second – represented here by Tay-Sachs's disease – the macular lesion is part of a generalized lipoid degeneration.

Doyne's Choroiditis The 'honeycomb choroiditis' of Doyne is characterized by the appearance of numerous colloid deposits between the optic disc and the macula. The condition is familial and is more often seen in women. The age of onset is in middle life and at first the colloid deposits do not interfere with vision. As the condition progresses, the deposits increase in size and extent and degenerative changes and haemorrhages occur in the retina. Central vision is then seriously affected. Fig. 1 shows the typical 'honeycomb' arrangement of the deposits.

Other Hereditary Degenerations A less well-defined familial degeneration is depicted in the drawings Figs 2 and 3, and the fundus photograph (Fig. 4). The changes have been grouped according to the period of life at which they become manifest into infantile, juvenile, adolescent, adult and senile types but the clinical picture is similar in them all. It is usual for all affected members of a family to develop the condition at the same age and for the nature of the lesion and its rate of progression to be similar in each family. In the senile group it is often difficult to obtain a family history and many of the cases usually described as simple senile changes at the macula may really be familial in type.

The presenting symptom is diminished visual acuity and a relative central scotoma can be elicited. As the disease advances, central vision is further reduced and may be completely abolished.

The macular lesion may be very slight initially and usually consists of a fine punctate stippling of pigment with small pale areas similar to colloid bodies. In Fig. 2 the exudate has conglomerated in the fovea and is surrounded by a pigmented ring. Fig. 3 is a drawing of the fundus of this patient's sister, showing the marked similarity of the changes.

The fundus photograph (Fig. 4) shows the left eye of a patient in whom the degeneration has progressed to such a degree that the macula appears as a hole through which the choroidal vessels can be clearly seen.

Familial Lipoid Degeneration This condition can be classified according to the age of onset but the pathology is essentially a primary lipoid degeneration of the ganglion cells of the entire nervous system, in which the ganglion cells of the retina are involved.

The most common form, Tay-Sachs's disease or amaurotic family idiocy, is confined to members of the Jewish race. Clinically the child is normal at birth but fails to develop normally and cannot sit or hold its head up, owing to weakness of the muscles of the neck and back. Finally it becomes completely paralysed and dies in a state of marasmus.

The ophthalmoscopic appearance will confirm the diagnosis, as the fundus picture seen in Fig. 5 is quite typical. It resembles that caused by acute obstruction of the central retinal artery, although the aetiology is altogether different. Around the macula is a white, somewhat raised area fading off into normal fundus at the periphery. At the centre of the white area the fovea shows clearly as a 'cherry-red' spot. Later, some degree of optic atrophy with narrowing of the vessels follows.

There is no treatment for the condition.

83

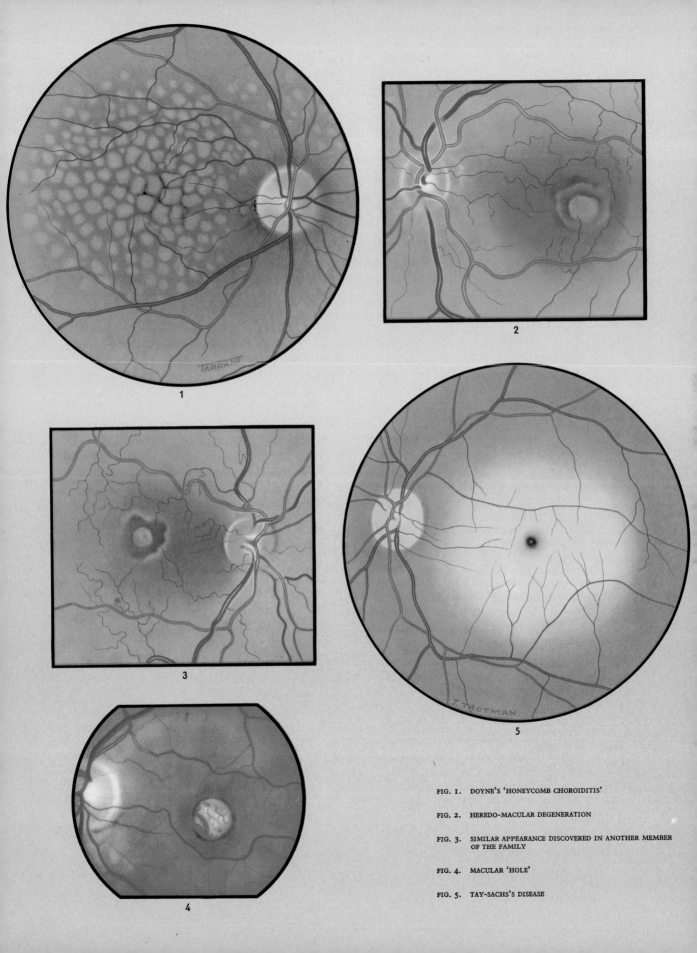

FIG. 1. DOYNE'S 'HONEYCOMB CHOROIDITIS'

FIG. 2. HEREDO-MACULAR DEGENERATION

FIG. 3. SIMILAR APPEARANCE DISCOVERED IN ANOTHER MEMBER OF THE FAMILY

FIG. 4. MACULAR 'HOLE'

FIG. 5. TAY-SACHS'S DISEASE

Senile Macular Degenerations

SENILE DEGENERATION at the macula is a common cause of reduced visual acuity in elderly patients and the early stages of these changes may be difficult to see until the pupil is dilated and the macula carefully examined.

Colloid Bodies Small well-defined yellowish spots are commonly found at the posterior pole in elderly patients. They are well illustrated in Fig. 1 and are due to the deposition of hyaline material in Bruch's membrane. Fortunately they cause little visual disturbance in themselves and cases in which the vision does deteriorate are probably due to concurrent senile and sclerotic changes in the choroid.

Chorio-Retinal Degeneration The macula derives its blood supply almost entirely from the chorio-capillaris, and sclerotic degenerative changes in the latter will inevitably produce deterioration of the retina at this site. The first recognizable changes are pigment disturbances and loss of the foveal reflex. Central vision is affected early and as the degeneration progresses so the visual acuity diminishes until the patient is unable to read.

The disease starts in one eye but soon becomes bilateral and the slow steady progression may be complicated by haemorrhages from the retina or choroid. Yellowish patches of exudate remain after such haemorrhages have been absorbed. Fig. 2 shows a typical senile macula – pigment disturbances and ill-defined exudates can be seen. The hard yellow streak of exudate in Fig. 1 is probably the end-result of a small haemorrhage.

Treatment is unlikely to stay the course of the lesion but optical aids may enable the remaining vision to be used to the best advantage.

Central Choroidal Sclerosis This is really an extension of the previous condition in which the choroidal sclerosis has advanced to such a degree that the capillary layer has vanished and the sclerosed choroidal vessels can be seen clearly through the depigmented retina (Fig. 3). Central vision is necessarily severely reduced.

Circinate Degeneration Although this condition has been reported in young people it is primarily a disease of old age.

The clinical picture as shown in the drawing (Fig. 4) and the fundus photograph (Fig. 5) is striking. A ring of hard yellowish, confluent exudates surrounds the macula which also shows pigmentary degeneration.

The aetiology of the condition is somewhat obscure. The exudates may be the result of haemorrhages in the retina or may follow an acute oedematous condition. In Fig. 4 the changes followed an oedema of the central area and the circinate exudates appeared after the swelling had subsided, thus delineating the margins of the affected retina. The condition tends to progress and central vision is severely affected.

85

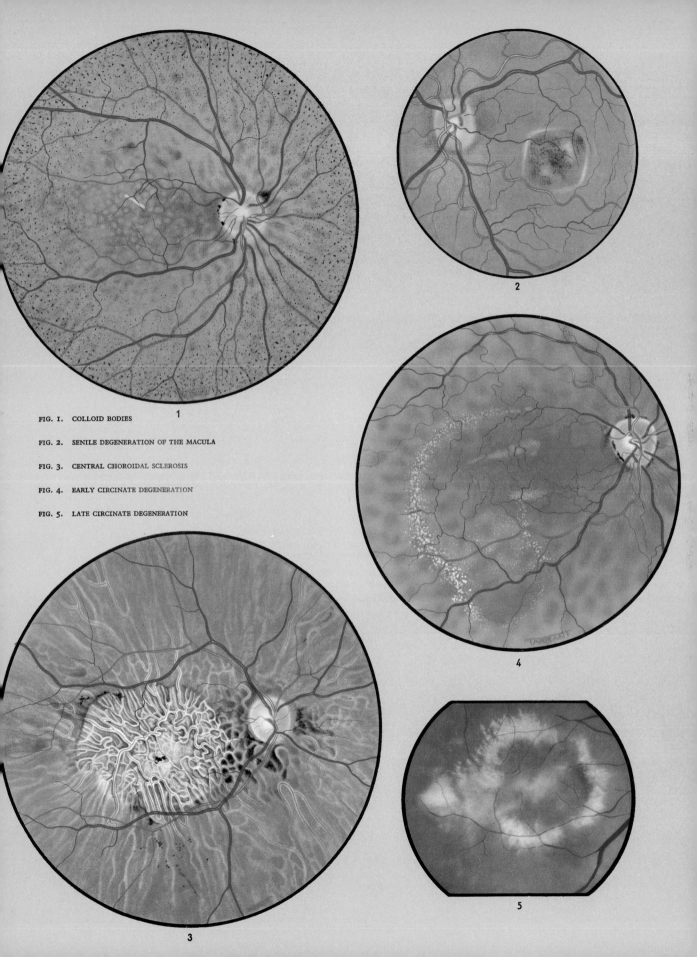

FIG. 1. COLLOID BODIES

FIG. 2. SENILE DEGENERATION OF THE MACULA

FIG. 3. CENTRAL CHOROIDAL SCLEROSIS

FIG. 4. EARLY CIRCINATE DEGENERATION

FIG. 5. LATE CIRCINATE DEGENERATION

Index

Index (cont.)

Index (cont.)

Index (cont.)

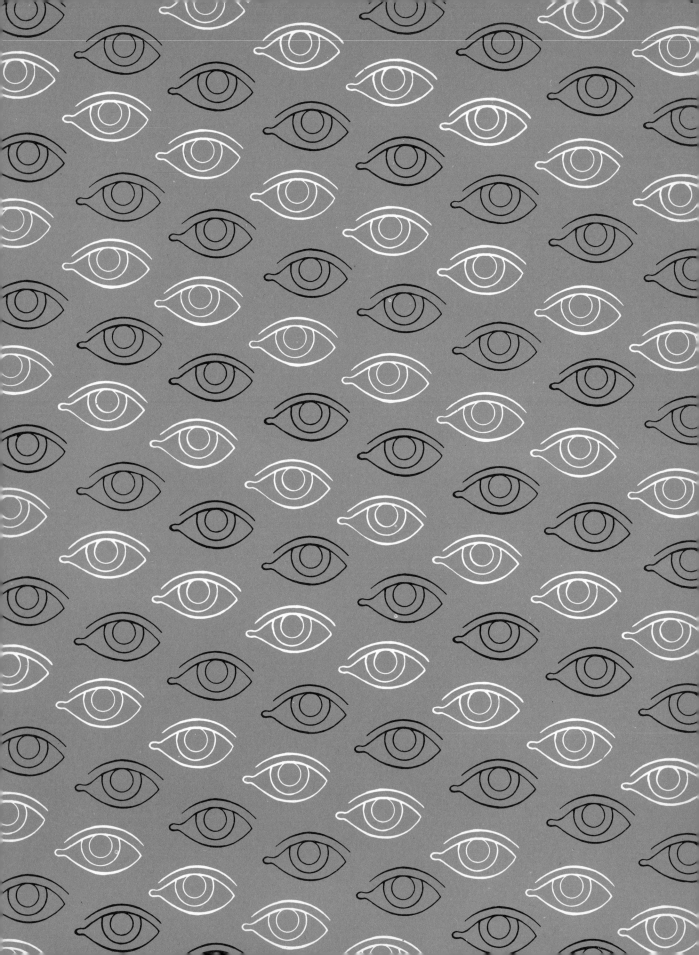